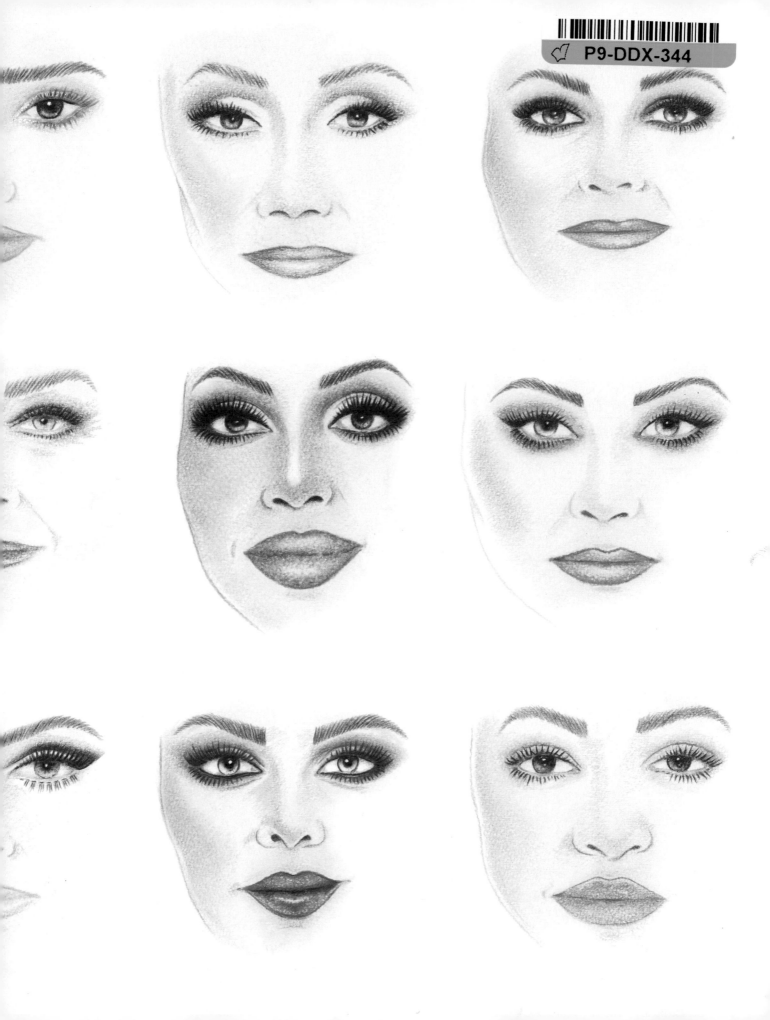

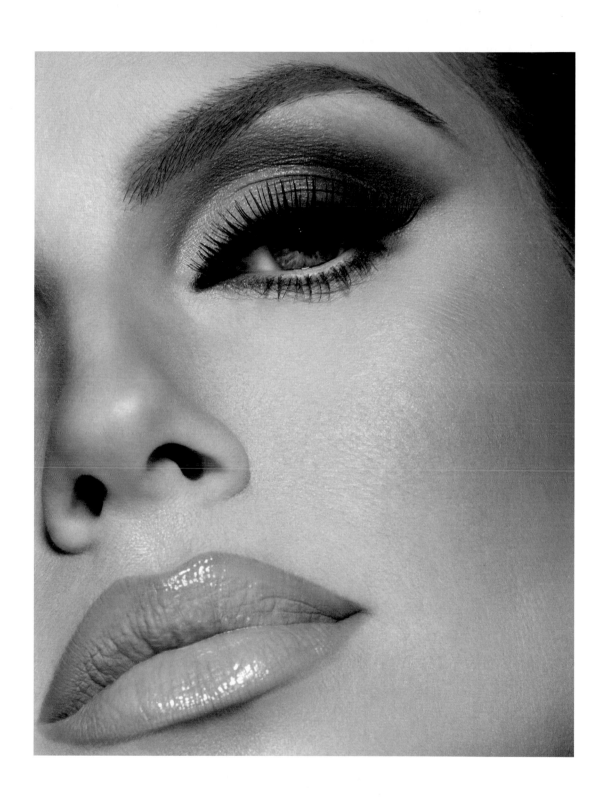

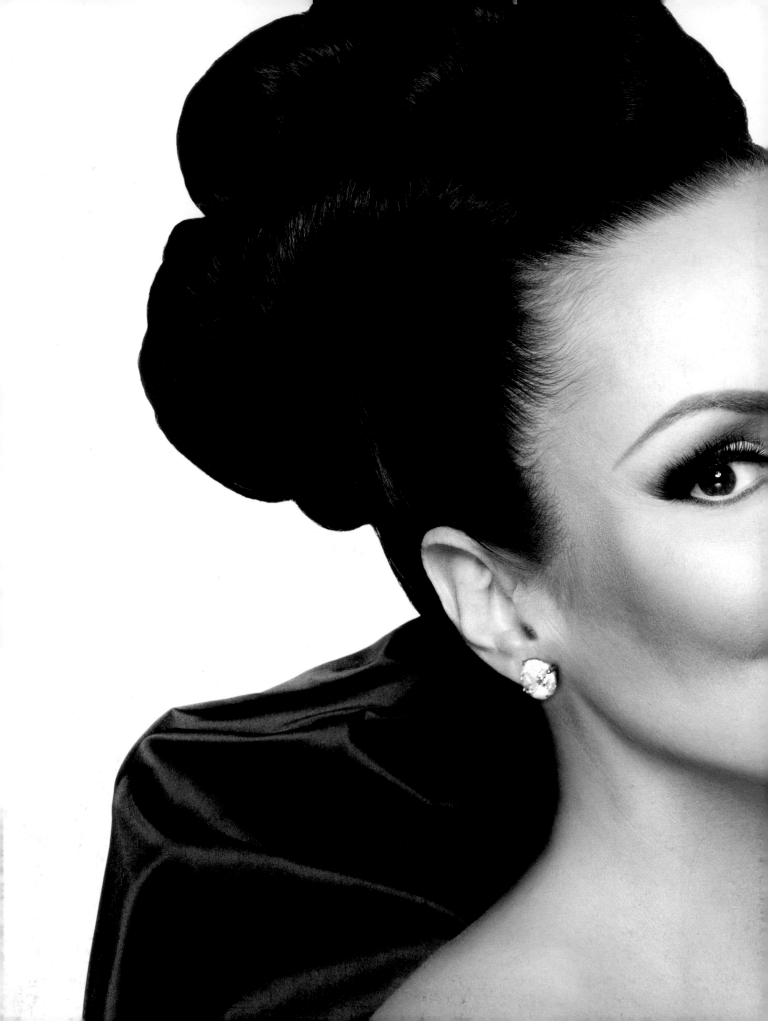

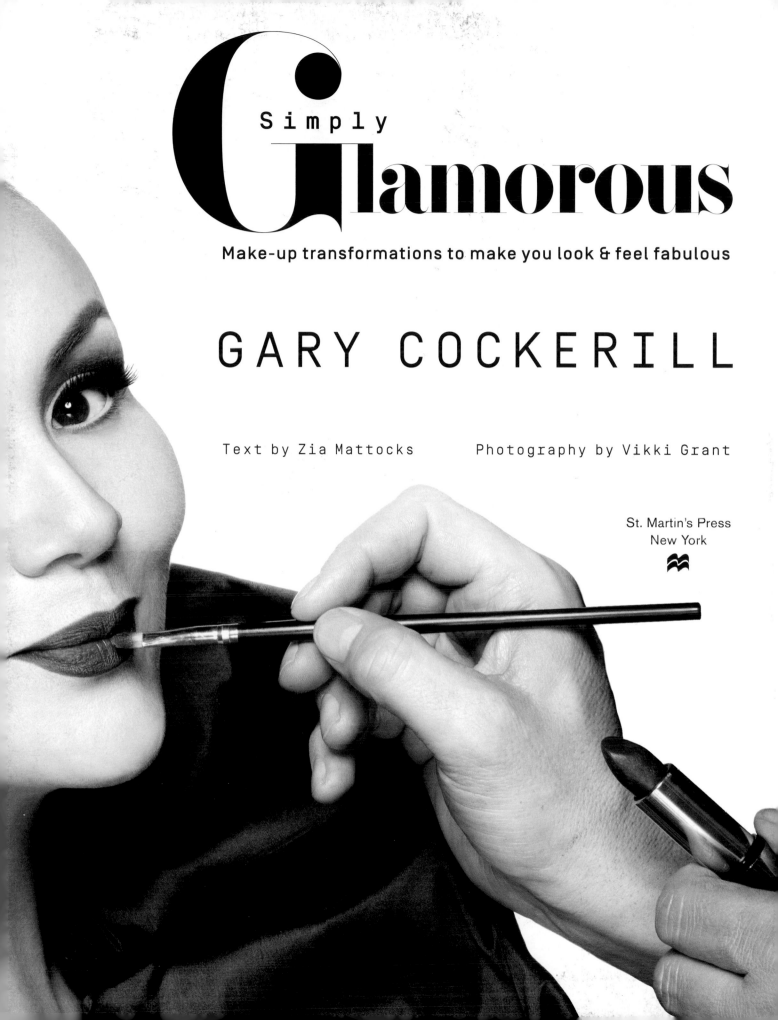

Simply Glamorous

Make-up transformations to make you look & feel fabulous

GARY COCKERILL

Text by Zia Mattocks   Photography by Vikki Grant

St. Martin's Press
New York

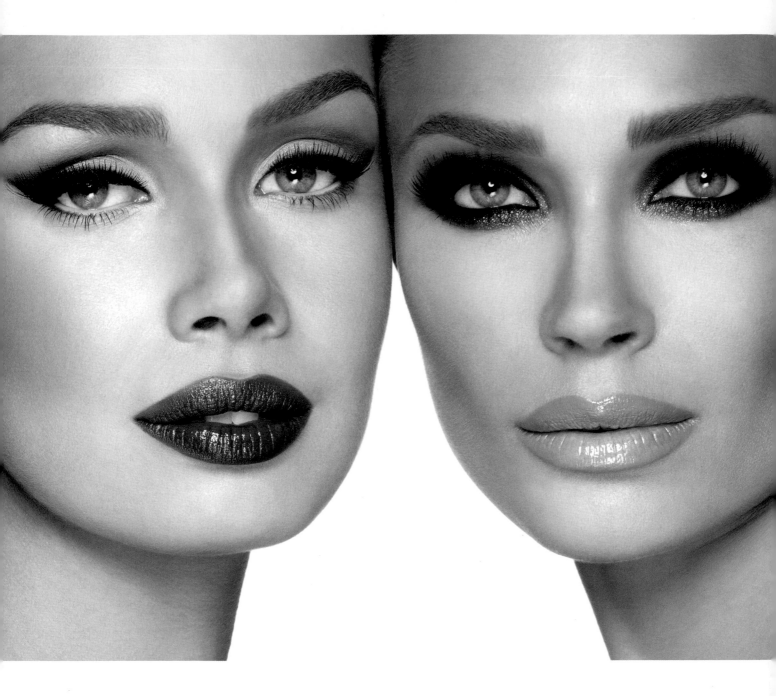

Printed in China.
For information, address
St. Martin's Press, 175 Fifth Avenue,
New York, N.Y. 10010.

www.stmartins.com

The written instructions, photographs,
designs, patterns, and projects in this
volume are intended for personal use
of the reader and may be reproduced
for that purpose only.

Library of Congress Cataloging-in-
Publication Data Available Upon Request

ISBN 978-1-250-07067-8

St. Martin's Press books may be
purchased for educational, business, or
promotional use. For information on bulk
purchases, please contact the Macmillan
Corporate and Premium Sales Department
at 1-800-221-7945, extension 5442, or
write to specialmarkets@macmillan.com.

First U.S. Edition: October 2015

10 9 8 7 6 5 4 3 2 1

*Transformations are
listed in italics*

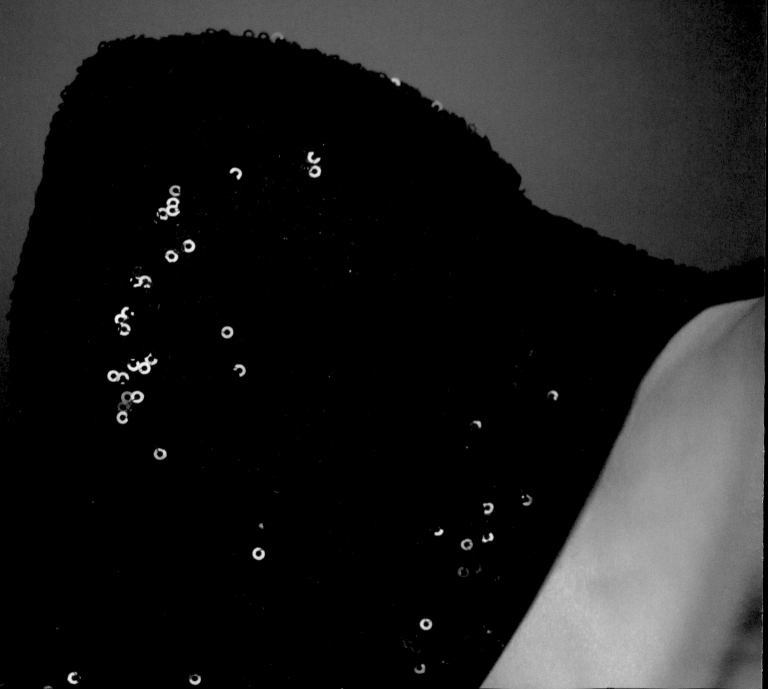

I could not have done this book without all
the wonderful women featured on the following
pages and around the world, who have touched
my life, inspired my ideas, defined my perceptions
of what beauty is, and proved that being simply
glamorous can change your life.

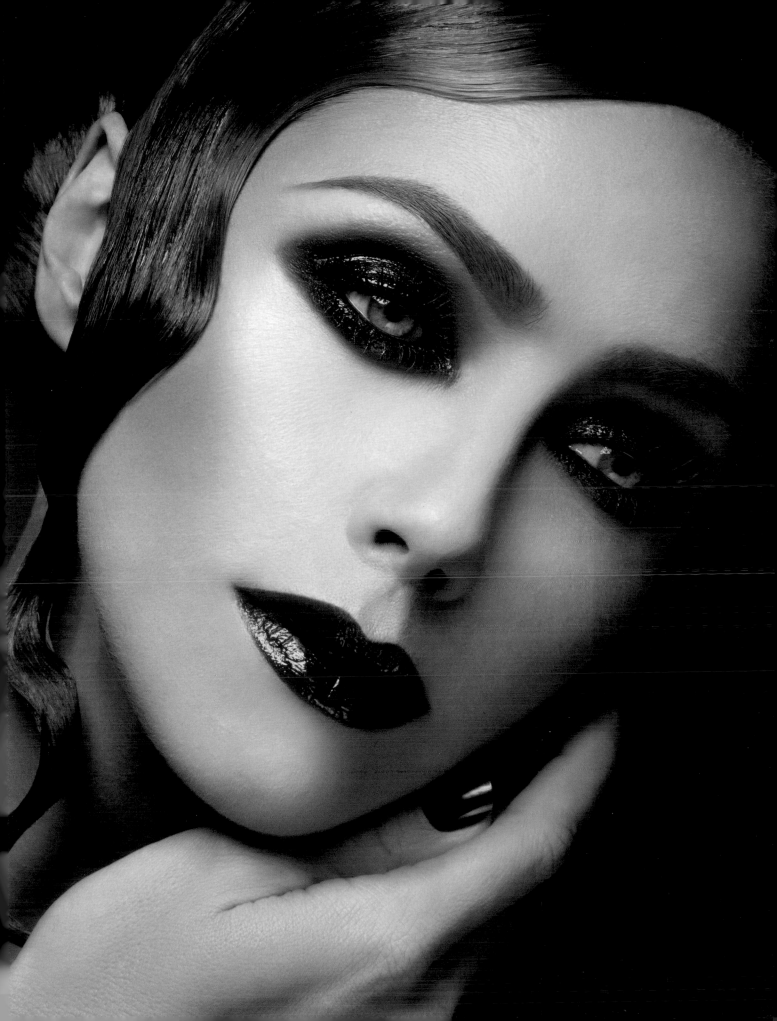

Introduction

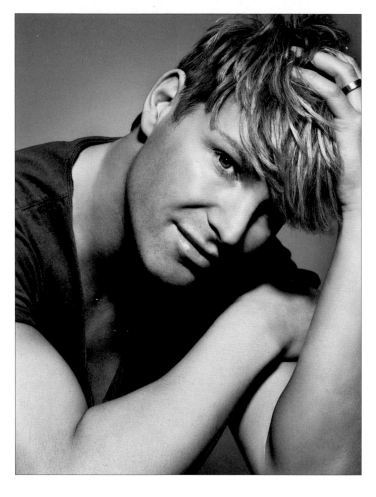

I often wonder, is beauty only skin deep? When I was about 22, I visited a psychic, who told me, "You're a healer." I had no idea what she meant and it took me years to understand that in many ways maybe I am. I create beauty with my hands; I give women confidence, which in turn helps them to achieve their goals in life; and I have the ability to transform and change the perception of how they think they should look, how they do look, and, more importantly, how they feel. People say that if you feel good on the inside, you look good on the outside. I agree, but looking great can also make you feel far stronger.

There is beauty in everyone, but we are often not able to see it in ourselves. We are all beautiful in our own way, but how do we find and enhance our own particular beauty? Look in the mirror and analyze yourself, remembering that age is just a number. What do you like about yourself and what would you change if you could? One of the things that drives and inspires me is the transformative power of make-up—and, in turn, the power a transformation can have on a person. When I make someone up, whether the make-up style is subtle, dramatic, timeless, or innovative, I am frequently amazed by how they seem to take on a new persona. Our ideas and perception of beauty are not always the same, but if I can help to reveal someone's beauty, then that's the best thing I can do and it's what makes my job worthwhile. I find that many people are afraid of make-up, but what is there to be afraid of? It's not complicated and if you don't like the results, it's easy to wash off and start again. Expressing yourself through the way you look gives you a certain kind of power and encourages a positive state of mind—everybody wants to look and feel beautiful.

As a child, I painted faces on any scrap of paper or surface I could find. I defaced all my parents' album covers, even adding lashes and lipstick to magazine covers when I thought I could make the person look more glamorous. I always had a love of the theater and movies and all the associated drama and glamour, and I was drawn to the strong female icons of the time who embodied everything I thought a beautiful woman should be. I would study their glamour, analyzing a face, picking it apart, and thinking about how I could improve it. Blank canvases were even better and I pleaded with my parents to buy me a Girl's World Styling Head. My sister soon became my muse and I would regularly beg her to let me transform her into my idols.

My passion was art and I excelled at it, but job opportunities for a working-class boy in Yorkshire, England, were limited and I decided I needed to find a way to make the move to a big city. It was the last year before England's mining industry started to decline and coal mines all over the north of the country began to be closed down. I saw an ad for work in the local pit and, much to my parents' dismay, I applied. It was hard, dirty work that was both physically and mentally draining, but it was a means to an end. I hated being in the bowels of the earth all day, but I admired the sense of camaraderie among the men.

After seven months, I had managed to stash away enough of my danger money to head to London to follow an as-yet-undefined dream. My parents thought I'd be back within the week but I was determined to make something of my life. I knew I wanted to do something art-related but I didn't know exactly what and I wasn't having much luck finding a job. That all changed when I saw an ad for an assistant to someone who painted shop mannequins. Getting that job was a stroke of pure luck, as that's where I learned about bone structure, definition, contouring, and the use of color and contrast. I saw how to paint a three-dimensional face and suddenly what I'd been drawing on paper for years was brought to life. When one of my friends asked me to do her make-up and we both loved the result, the idea of becoming a make-up artist dawned on me.

I hounded photographers and agents to give me unpaid "testing" work until, eventually, I started getting my own bookings. I was very fortunate to have met the right people at the right time. It was during the era when "heroin chic" was all over the catwalks and high-fashion magazines, and my make-up style was the polar opposite. I did a lot of work at the time for lifestyle magazines, as they wanted their cover girls to look glamorous and sexy, not pale and pasty. A lot of celebrities also seemed to want the high-impact looks that I began to be known for, and the bookings flooded in.

After working in the beauty industry for more than 25 years, I want to share my knowledge, expertise, and passion for creating beauty. I hope this book will inspire and educate, as well as give you the confidence to have fun with make-up and experiment with your look. I'm self-taught, so I'm not a textbook make-up artist, but the

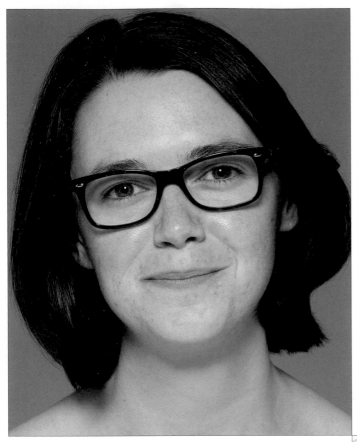

"I don't wear much make-up in everyday life—even when I go out—so it was a pretty dramatic transformation. I thought I was almost unrecognizable! It was amazing and definitely showed me what is possible."

I always start a makeover by analyzing the person's bare face and seeing how I can make the most of it—what I can enhance, improve, or play down—or just how I can make my client look different and, above all, feel good about herself. Charlotte hardly ever wears make-up and has never really experimented with it, so I wanted to demonstrate how transformative it can be. The look had to have a real "Wow!" factor, focusing on her beautiful eyes that are contoured to make them appear larger and framed with perfect, Elizabeth Taylor-style arched brows. The glamorous look is completed with apricot cream blush, defining the cheeks, and creamy nude lips that don't steal the limelight.

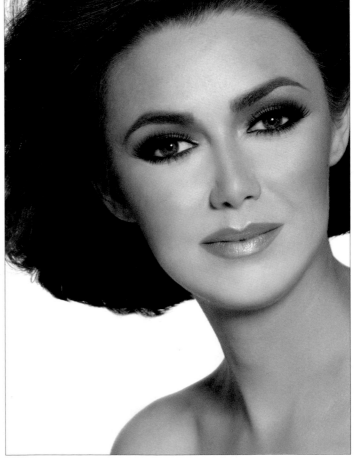

techniques I use work for me and achieve the results I want. In my view, there's no real right or wrong way with make-up—it's about experimenting and making make-up work for you. I do what I feel is right; I tailor the make-up first and foremost to the person, and then to the look and mood that we want to create. One of my favorite aspects of my work is the different people I meet. I love talking to women and I really listen to what they want, which makes them feel comfortable, and then it becomes easy for me to work with them to create a look that makes them feel beautiful.

On the following pages, I've aimed to demonstrate the art of make-up and its power of illusion, but also to prove how accessible it is and how many looks that appear complicated are actually relatively easy to achieve. The looks I've demonstrated are there as a guideline and a springboard— some colors and tones may not be for you, but you don't need to copy exactly what I've done. You can take elements you like, change the colors or textures, leave off the false lashes, or add more. I've just shown you a couple of ways of interpreting a look, and if they spark a single idea, make you completely re-evaluate your look, or inspire you to open your make-up bag and throw away all the old products you've had in there for 10 or 20 years, then this book has done its job.

I've chosen a collection of looks that I hope will appeal to the widest audience. They're all ones that I'm often asked to create—some are contemporary takes on the classics, some are subtle and natural, while others are more extreme, often pushing the boundaries with the use of color and texture. I have carried them out on a wonderful range of women, of all ages and ethnicities, some who rarely wear make-up, some who have no idea how to wear make-up, some who have always

wanted to try new looks but have never had the confidence, and others who like to experiment but were happy to learn some new techniques. I painted a bespoke face chart for each person that sums up the finished look I created for them, with a list of all the make-up colors and textures I used. Every face and every personality is different, and I would love you to try out some new products, tricks, and techniques, and adapt the looks you like to work for you. As a former coal miner turned make-up artist, I'm living proof that rules can be broken, so don't let anything hold you back from showing the world your beauty and feeling fabulous.

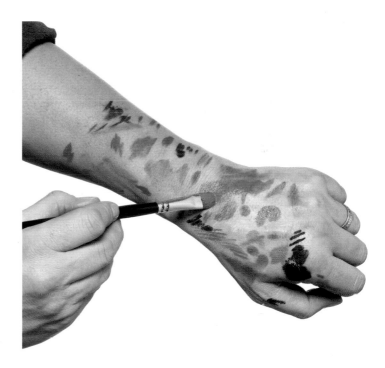

One face four ways

The lovely Kelly Brook has the perfect face for showcasing how transformative make-up can be. She's classically beautiful but, as an actress, she's also a chameleon. Often make-up artists advise that dramatic eyes should be offset with low-key lips, and vice versa. I believe it depends on how you apply the make-up and how much your face can take—as well as the occasion—so I wanted to demonstrate four key looks that anyone can wear. Try all combinations, as what you think won't work might actually suit you best.

1 Neutral eyes & lips

I contoured her face with two shades of cream foundation to create a flawless complexion. I defined her brows with a brow powder one shade lighter than her hair, and swept an apricot eyeshadow into her socket and under the lower lash line at the outer edge of her eyes. I added a few lash clusters to the outer edge and mid-section of the upper lash line; with a coat of mascara, this dressed up the eyes just enough. The lipstick is neutral and tones with the eyes, with a touch of gloss to bring them alive. I added apricot blush to warm up her cheeks, with champagne highlighter along the cheekbones for a youthful sheen.

2 Dark eyes & light lips

As before, the face is creamy and flawless, and the brows are softly defined. I blended a darker, toning shadow into the socket line and outer corner of the eye, keeping the focus on the upper lid. I used a gel liner along the upper lash line, keeping it fine at the beginning of the eye, slightly thickening it from the mid-section onward, and flicking it up at the end. I added a few more lash clusters and mascara on the roots and lower lashes. To counterbalance the drama on the eyes, I chose a light, soft lip color that tones with the skin—I outlined the lips with a beige-pink lip pencil and filled them in, keeping them matte and understated.

3 Light eyes & dark lips

The key to this make-up is to have perfectly arched brows to frame the understated eyes. I applied a skin-tone colored eyeshadow over the lid and up to the brow bone and emphasized the socket with a warm taupe. I then applied black gel liner to her upper lash line, keeping the line quite minimal with a slight flick at the end. I filled in the lashes with a few individual and cluster lashes, and applied mascara to the roots. All the drama is on the lips, which I lined and contoured with a deep scarlet lip liner and then filled in with a slightly lighter red lipstick. The result is beautiful matte lips with a velvety finish.

4 Dark eyes & dark lips

With heavy make-up on the eyes and lips, I used a light foundation to keep the skin natural rather than mask-like. The brows are soft and neatly arched. I applied a charcoal eyeshadow to the main part of the eyelid and blended it outward, creating a smoky effect. I lined the lash lines and waterlines with black kohl pencil to build up the intensity. I used individual and cluster lashes, but you can leave these off if you feel they'd overwhelm the look—a coat or two of mascara may be all you need. To accentuate Kelly's lips, I lined them with a dark berry pencil and built up the color with a slightly lighter berry-red satin lipstick.

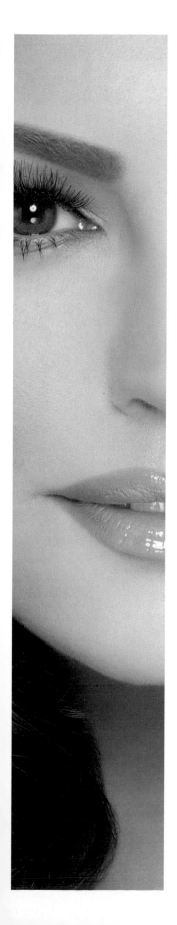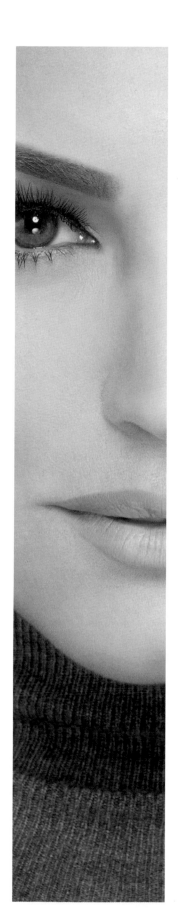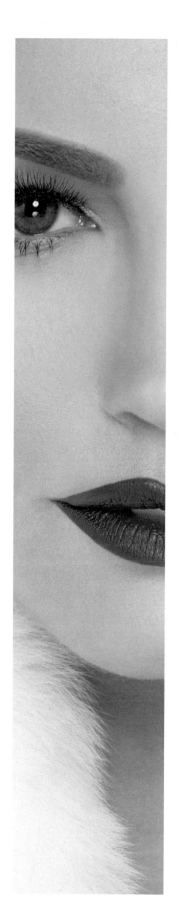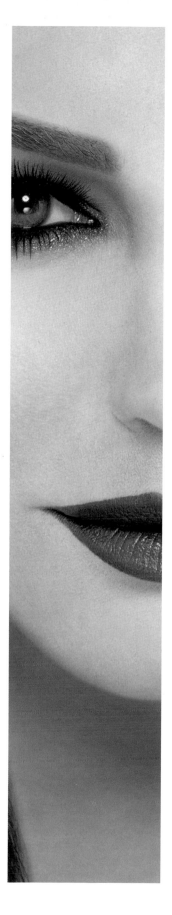

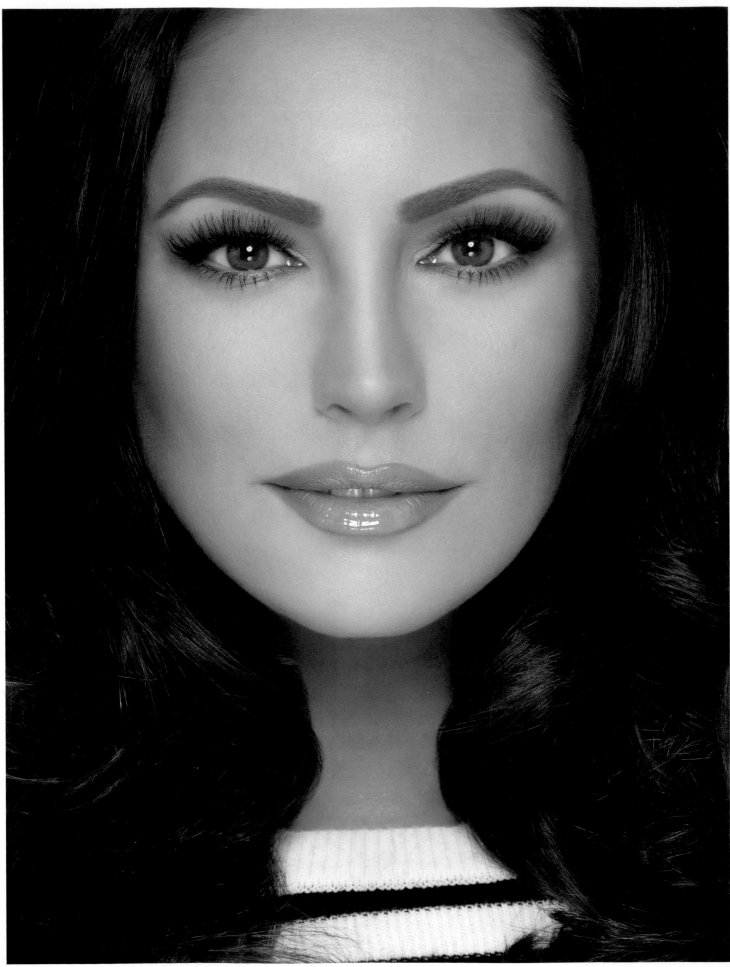

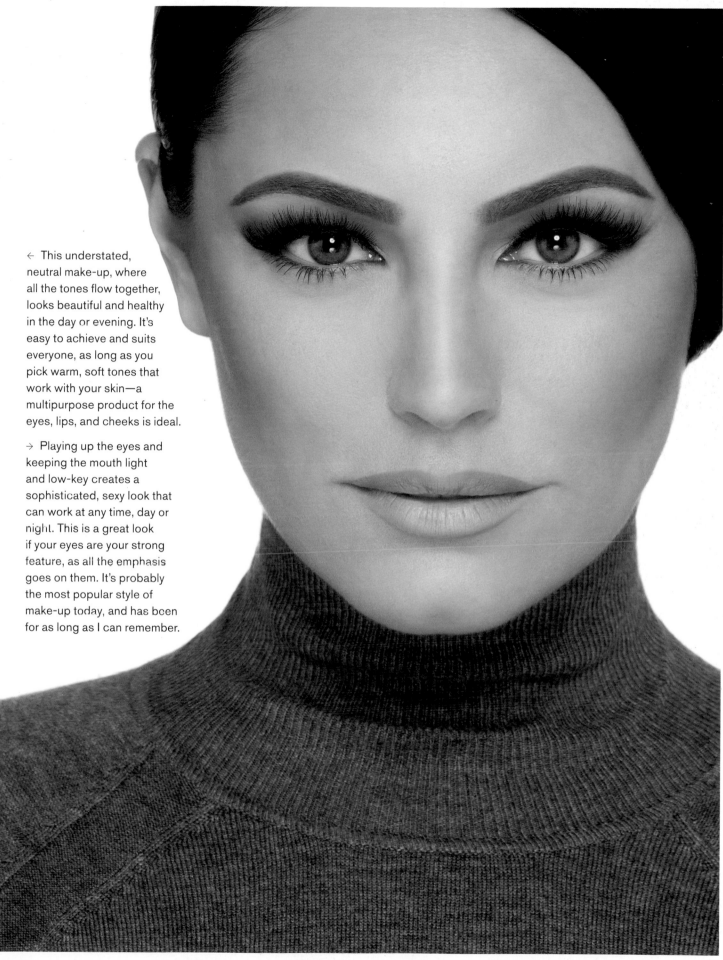

← This understated, neutral make-up, where all the tones flow together, looks beautiful and healthy in the day or evening. It's easy to achieve and suits everyone, as long as you pick warm, soft tones that work with your skin—a multipurpose product for the eyes, lips, and cheeks is ideal.

→ Playing up the eyes and keeping the mouth light and low-key creates a sophisticated, sexy look that can work at any time, day or night. This is a great look if your eyes are your strong feature, as all the emphasis goes on them. It's probably the most popular style of make-up today, and has been for as long as I can remember.

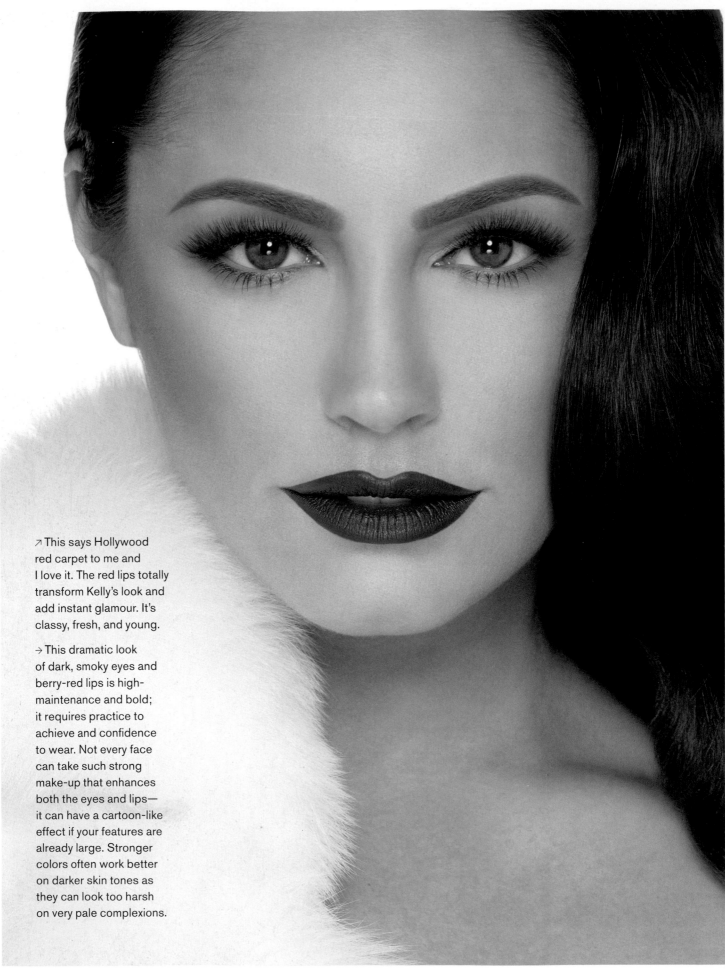

↗ This says Hollywood red carpet to me and I love it. The red lips totally transform Kelly's look and add instant glamour. It's classy, fresh, and young.

→ This dramatic look of dark, smoky eyes and berry-red lips is high-maintenance and bold; it requires practice to achieve and confidence to wear. Not every face can take such strong make-up that enhances both the eyes and lips— it can have a cartoon-like effect if your features are already large. Stronger colors often work better on darker skin tones as they can look too harsh on very pale complexions.

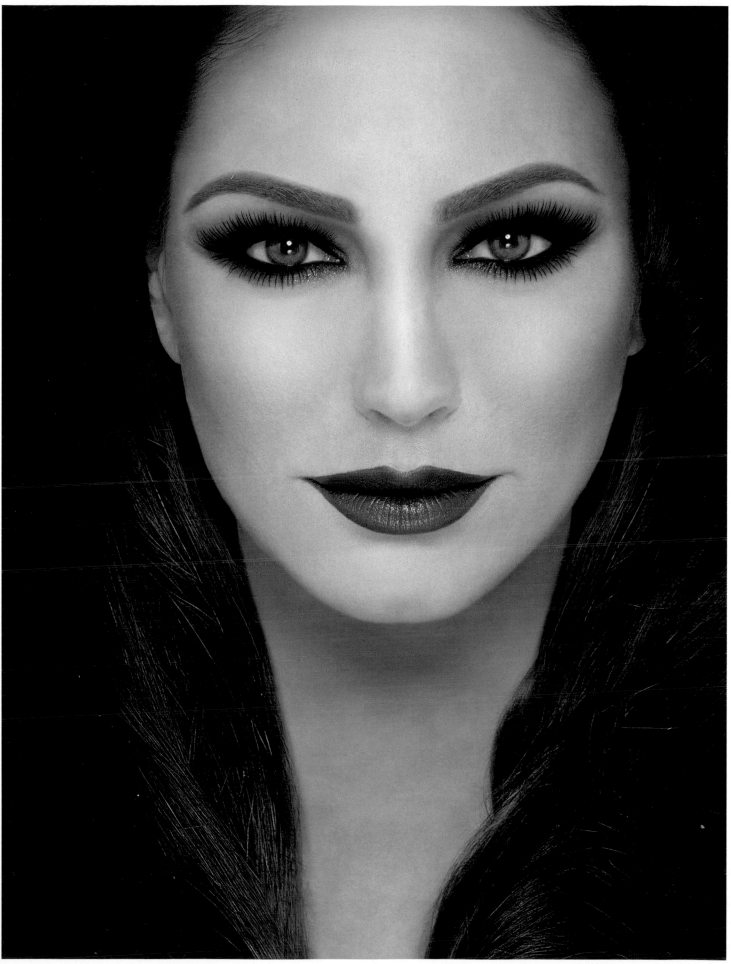

gary's guide to gorgeous

1
There are no rules. Less is more; more is more. Individuality is the greatest gift we have and make-up is a great way to showcase this and exercise creativity and self-expression.

2
It's all about balance. Too much of one thing or not enough of something else can make or break a look. When you're deciding what make-up look to apply, analyze the shape of your eyes and lips and decide which area you want to draw attention to. Try to assess your make-up objectively, taking your whole outfit into account, to ensure you look and feel gorgeous.

3
Don't get stuck in a rut. The make-up you wore when you were 21 won't look right when you're 51. Regularly go through your make-up bag and chuck out old products—and don't be afraid to try out new ones. Be inspired, borrow ideas, use references. We've all been there and done it before—style and fashion comes around, so let it inspire you, draw from it, and make it your own.

4
Give yourself enough time. Whether you are doing a 5-minute or a 35-minute make-up look, you have to blend, blend, blend to create a perfect finish. If you cut corners, the result won't look as good. Natural light and artificial light are very different, so make sure your make-up looks good in whichever you are going to be seen. Daylight is less forgiving, so natural make-up usually looks better—save the full-on dramatic looks for the evening.

5

Hygiene is so important. I read somewhere that a make-up bag can harbor more bacteria than a toilet. Always wash your hands before you apply your make-up and clean your brushes and sponges afterward. Wash your make-up bag regularly and always put the tops back on things.

6

Be creative. There are always ways to adapt a look to make it work for you. If you don't like the color combinations, try different ones; if you think false lashes will be too much for you, just wear mascara; if you don't want matte lips, choose a satin finish instead.

7

Be brave. Don't dismiss a color, texture, or look until you try it. You may be surprised to discover that something you always thought would never suit you actually looks fantastic.

8

Don't forget your body. If other parts of your body are going to be on show, try to tie them in to the look—perhaps a touch of fake tan on your arms, a dusting of shimmery highlighter on your collarbone.

9

Do you get what you pay for? You can spend extortionate amounts on make-up but often you don't need to. The result you get from make-up has more to do with how you apply it than its price tag. No matter how much you spend, it won't look good if you don't know how to put it on, so you're wasting your money. There are many good inexpensive products, but do test them to make sure they contain enough pigment. Instead of buying expensive make-up brushes, go to an art shop and get them for a quarter of the price, and try multipurpose products that save you time and money.

10

Love yourself. This is the most important thing, because if you don't, it can affect everything from your confidence and your sexuality to the image you project and how you look. Don't lose sight of your unique natural beauty— there are so many ways you can play up your good features, so don't become someone else.

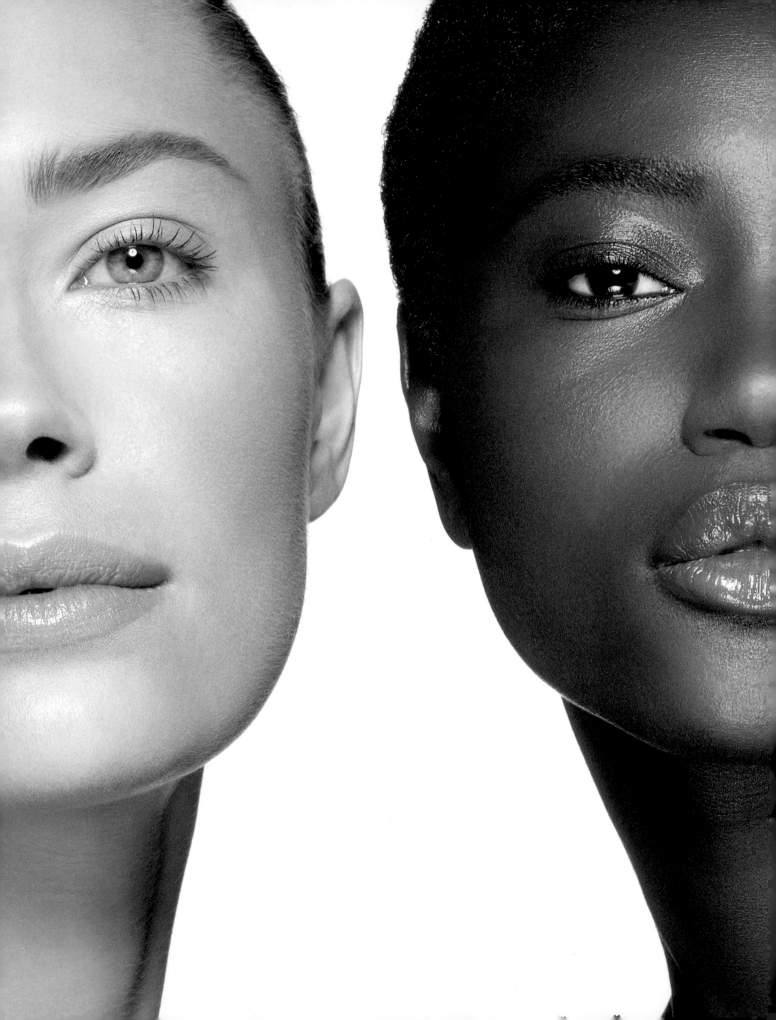

face

Everyone's face is
unique—the color
and texture of your
skin, the shape of
your face, and your
features. None of
these remains constant
throughout the course
of your life—the
seasons, hormonal
fluctuations, diet,
lifestyle, and the
aging process all
have an effect—so
I suggest that you
assess your face
fairly regularly to
see whether you could
change the way you
go about enhancing
it. Your face is your
canvas and there are
many ways to paint it.

Healthy Skin

The skin is an amazing organ—and the largest in the body. It allows us to feel the sensation of touch, provides a physical barrier against the environment, helps to control our body temperature, and to eliminate toxins through perspiration. So aside from our desire to look good, it's also in our body's interest to take care of our skin and ensure it's as healthy as it can be.

Good genes certainly help, but good skincare can go a long way to giving you beautiful, radiant skin that glows with health. There are a number of environmental and lifestyle factors that can affect the condition of your skin, such as exposure to the sun, extreme cold, and pollution, and what you eat, how much you exercise, the quality of your sleep, and how much stress you're under.

I'm not a dermatologist but I know that the skin needs nourishment and nurturing to keep it functioning at its optimum. If we are healthy on the inside and give our body the nutrients it requires, this will reflect in our skin. Many people find that if they are sensitive to certain food types—dairy or wheat products, for example—their skin will suffer from breakouts, inflammation, eczema, or other skin conditions. If this is you, it stands to reason you will try to avoid those foods, and if the problem persists, I always recommend going to see a doctor or dermatologist who can identify the cause and advise on the best course of treatment.

The skin constantly renews and rejuvenates itself, shedding old skin cells and replacing them with new ones. Nutrients are essential to support this process, to strengthen the capillaries that convey them around the body, and to stimulate the production of collagen, which gives the skin its elasticity—and sadly diminishes as we age, leading to wrinkles and sagging. Key skin-supporting vitamins are Vitamins A, B, C, D, E, and K.

Also vital—both for our general health and for helping to slow down the aging process—are antioxidants, which neutralize the unstable free radicals found in the atmosphere. Antioxidants include some of the vitamins mentioned and are found in many fruits and vegetables, especially the so-called "superfoods," such as berries and kale. Essential fatty acids, such as Omega-3 and Omega-6, found in oily fish, avocados, and eggs, keep the skin supple and help to reduce inflammation. Sugar, animal fat, alcohol, and processed foods are all damaging to the skin in large quantities and should, ideally, be avoided.

Tips for healthy skin

There are lots of simple ways to help your
skin stay healthy, hydrated, free from
breakouts, and looking as youthful as
possible for as long as possible.
Once you understand your own skin
and how it behaves, it's easy
to get into a good routine
that will ensure your
skin always looks
and feels great.

1 **Use sunscreen** and be very sensible about exposing your skin to the sun. Good facial sunscreens are now widely available and are incorporated in many moisturizers, primers, foundations, and lipsticks. Choose one that protects against both UVA and UVB rays.

2 **Don't smoke.** As well as all the other associated health issues, smoking is bad for the skin. It makes it look dull and accelerates the signs of aging by destroying collagen and causing lines and wrinkles.

3 **Eat well,** including lots of fresh, low-sugar, antioxidant-rich fruit and vegetables (such as blueberries and broccoli), as well as "good" fats found in oily fish, avocados, and almonds. Limit your intake of sugar, which is one of the biggest enemies of collagen.

Keep hydrated by drinking at least eight glasses of water a day. Avoid sugary drinks or anything containing additives.

4 **Exercise** increases blood flow, which carries nutrients and oxygen around the body.

5 **Get your beauty sleep.** Lack of sleep makes the skin dull and can create puffy eyes and dark circles.

6 **Moisturize**, moisturize, moisturize.

Cleanse your face well. Always take your make-up off before bed.

Wash your brushes and sponges after every application and take note of the shelf life printed on product packaging—make-up is a breeding ground for bacteria.

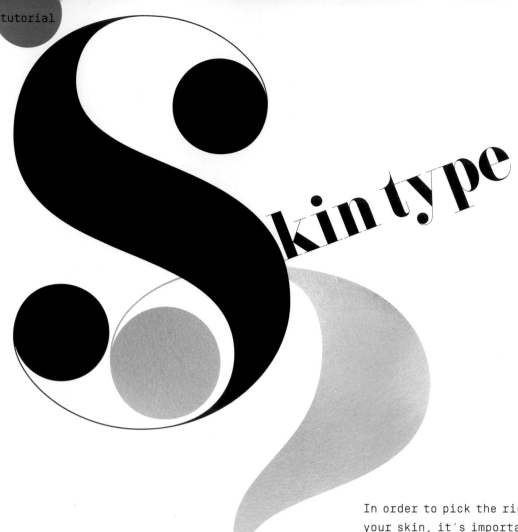

Skin type

In order to pick the right products to use on your skin, it's important to know your skin type. Using unsuitable products can lead to dryness and flakiness or, conversely, to an excess of sebum, the skin's natural oil, which may result in clogged pores and breakouts. It can also cause sensitivity or inflammation.

What's right for one person may not be right for another, but, as a general rule, I advise my clients to look for products that are rich in Vitamin E and free from fragrance and color. The other advice I give is to keep things simple. We are easily seduced by beauty editorials or enthusiastic sales staff and often buy things we don't necessarily need and end up putting too much on the skin.

Getting to know your skin is essential for creating the right skincare routine for you. Try to "listen" to your skin and pick products that suit it and give good results, remembering that this may change due to factors such as stress and aging. What might have been your skin type when you were younger can sometimes change for a variety of reasons—diet, hormones, environment, lifestyle, and so on. Consider the season as well, as you often need to change your products accordingly—from using richer moisturizer in the winter, to combat extreme cold and the drying effects of central heating, to swapping your foundation for a deeper shade in the summer months.

what type?

In the morning, wipe your face with a clean tissue. Normal or dry skin—the tissue will be clean. Oily skin—there will be an oily residue. Combination skin—there will be oil from the central part of the face (the T-zone of forehead, nose, and chin). Look at your skin in good light. Dry/dehydrated skin—looks dry with fine lines on the cheeks and feels tight or itchy. Very dry skin—there are dry, flaky patches. Sensitive skin—there are areas of redness or inflammation and the skin feels itchy.

dry

This type of skin usually looks dull and lacks luster and elasticity. There are often patches of dryness and visible fine lines. Eat a diet rich in essential fatty acids, fish oils, and Vitamin E. Use mild, hydrating cleansers, a rich day moisturizer with SPF, a hydrating serum, and a thick, creamy night cream to help seal in moisture. Look for moisturizing, hydrating foundations and choose creamy blushes rather than powder products.

oily

A shiny complexion with large pores indicates oily skin, which is prone to blocked pores, resulting in blackheads or blemishes. Excess sebum may be due to a hormonal imbalance, as well as factors such as stress or humidity. Choose calming products that are formulated to reduce oiliness. A mild exfoliator or deep-cleansing mask will help unblock pores. Choose powder-based products to counteract the oiliness, and matte finishes that won't highlight any blemishes.

combination

Most people have dry, normal, and oily areas, which may change through the seasons and as you age. The T-zone is often oily and there are sometimes dry patches on the cheeks. A foaming face wash will keep oily areas at bay without being too drying, but if your skin feels tight, use a cream cleanser at night and rich moisturizer on the dry areas. The aim is to balance the skin, so make sure your diet includes sufficient nutrients, especially Vitamins A, C, E, zinc, and selenium.

normal

This is the skin we'd all love to have. It's well balanced, so it's neither dry, nor oily, nor sensitive. It has a lot of elasticity and so it looks plump, glowing, and hydrated, with few imperfections and fine lines, and smaller pores. To keep it looking radiant, make sure you cleanse, tone, and moisturize on a daily basis. Use a gentle exfoliator once or twice a week to help slough away the dead skin cells and promote renewal, and always wear sunscreen.

sensitive

Sensitive skin is the most delicate skin type, which is readily prone to irritation, itching, redness, and flaky patches. Notice when a flair-up occurs and try to pinpoint the culprit—it could be something you've eaten or a new product you've applied. In general, choose skincare and make-up products that are specially formulated for sensitive skin and avoid those that contain perfumes, colorants, alcohol, or emulsifiers that might cause inflammation or irritation.

aging

The regeneration of skin cells slows as we age and the skin thins. It also dries, as sebaceous glands produce less lubricating sebum, making the surface look dull and lackluster. Collagen and fatty tissue break down, so the skin loses elasticity and plumpness, and starts to sag and wrinkle. Smoking and exposure to UVA rays accelerate this. Cream foundation is a good choice but avoid powdery products. Less is not always more, so don't be afraid to experiment.

Prep & prime

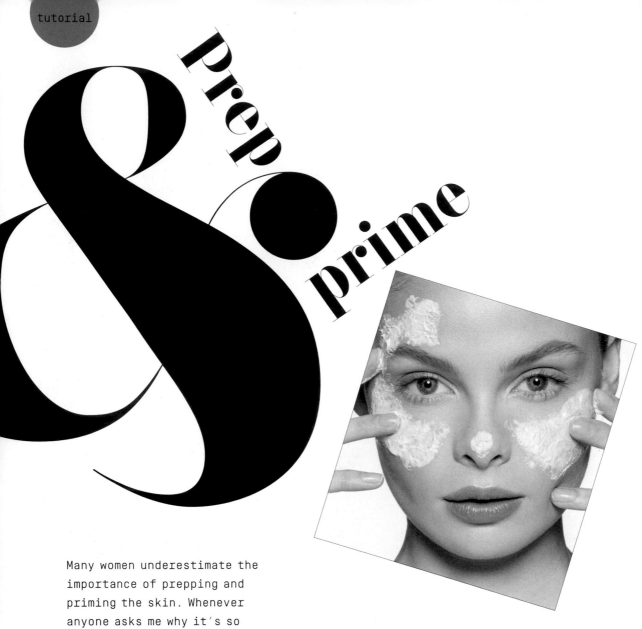

Many women underestimate the importance of prepping and priming the skin. Whenever anyone asks me why it's so important or whether it's something they can skip, I always tell them to think about when they're decorating their home. If you don't prepare your surfaces before you start, the wallpaper and paint won't stick and the finish won't be good. It's the same with your face.

cleanse

A freshly cleansed face looks radiant and glowing, but the skin can play host to lots of bacteria, so keeping it clean is essential to prevent breakouts and infections. Cleansing the face morning and evening is a must for everyone, but you may need to do it more depending on your occupation and lifestyle. The skin on your face is much thinner and more delicate and sensitive than the rest of your body, so it needs special care. Cleansers come in a wide variety of formats—from quick-fix wipes (best for occasional use) to creams, balms, gels, mousses, and oils. Choose one that's appropriate for your skin type and follow it up with toner and a targeted serum, if you wish, and a suitable moisturizer. Gel and foam are good choices for oily skin, while cream and oil are moisturizing for dry skin. Soap is a big no-no, as it strips the skin of its natural oils and dries it out. Don't scrub at the skin, but work in gentle, circular, massaging movements, sweeping your fingers up and outward to stimulate circulation and aid lymphatic drainage. Rinse well and then blot your face gently with a towel to dry.

exfoliate

Gentle exfoliation—whether with a washcloth, brush, cream, lotion, or granular scrub—polishes the skin and removes the dead skin cells that make the complexion look flat and dull. But don't overdo it, as too much exfoliation with too harsh a product will make the skin dry and could cause irritation or sensitivity—exfoliating once to three times a week is average, but everyone's skin is different.

tone

Whether you use toner is a personal choice. It leaves the skin feeling soothed, refreshed, and super-clean and is great for oily skin, as it removes excess oil and closes pores, but some people find it too drying. Many toners contain active ingredients that are antibacterial and anti-inflammatory, so choose one that's right for your skin type and avoid alcohol-based toners that tend to strip the skin of its natural oils.

moisturize

Essential for hydrating the skin and keeping the surface smooth and supple, moisturizer is the skincare staple. Whether a lotion, cream, or oil, moisturizer contains a variety of active ingredients to help slow down the aging process and nourish and protect the skin. Day cream tends to be light and readily absorbed, and often incorporates sunscreen. Night cream usually has a thicker consistency and is designed to aid the skin's renewal process while you sleep. Eye creams are specially formulated for the more delicate skin around the eyes. Oils are great for very dry skin and can be used alone or under cream, while concentrated serums are able to deliver their active ingredients to the deeper layers of the skin.

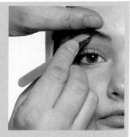

making good

Before beginning any makeover, the first thing I do is prepare the face. This is time well spent and makes all the difference to the quality of the finished make-up and its staying power.

After cleansing, toning, and moisturizing (see left), the next thing to do is set about removing any facial hair. This could just mean tweezing away the odd stray hair from the eyebrows to achieve a good, neat frame for the face (see page 96). Facial hair can be dealt with by cream, laser, electrolysis, waxing, threading, or bleaching. Excessive facial hair may be caused by a hormonal imbalance that can be treated medically, so ask your doctor about this and don't suffer in silence.

Face masks are great way to deep-cleanse and give your skin a boost. They stimulate the blood flow and refresh the complexion while drawing out impurities, exfoliating, or hydrating. A face mask can perk up tired, dull skin that's in need of a pick-me-up. Similarly, eye drops are a great way to brighten and whiten tired, red eyes.

PRIMERS

Available as cream, gel, or serum, primer creates a great base for make-up, filling in fine lines and pores and giving the skin a smoother finish. It ensures foundation glides on easily and improves its coverage and staying power. Primer may be formulated to moisturize, hydrate, illuminate, or absorb excess oil and mattify. They can be water-based or silicone-based. Some are tinted, pearlized, or light-reflective. They may be rich in antioxidants and anti-aging ingredients or designed to soothe irritation and minimize redness. Eye primers make eyeshadow last longer and ensure colors are true. Mascara primers, which are usually colorless, thicken and lengthen the lashes. Lip primers smooth the lips and increase the longevity of the lipstick.

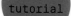
Correct and conceal

Most people suffer from blemishes and imperfections from time to time, but luckily there are some clever products on the market to help us deal with them and make them less noticeable. I am often asked if there's a difference between color correctors and concealers, and whether color correctors are really necessary. It's a simple answer: there's a big difference and, yes, by incorporating color correctors into your make-up routine, you can not only cover up an area but neutralize it too, and ensure your make-up holds its color and disguises any flaws.

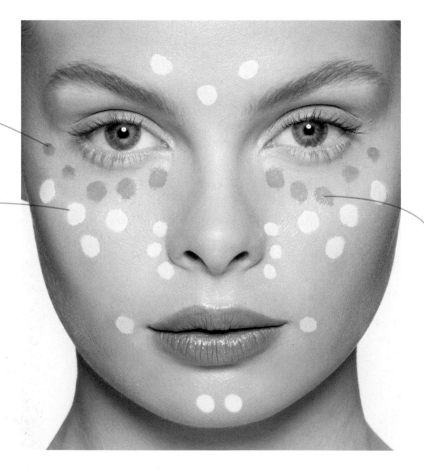

lilac *A pick-me-up that brightens the skin and counteracts dull, sallow tones.*

green *Cancels out redness, so good for covering rosacea, pimples, and broken capillaries on the cheeks or chin or around the nose. Light green or yellow is ideal for fair skin but if your skin is darker, choose a deeper shade to suit.*

peachy pink *Brightens the area under the eyes, masking signs of fatigue on fair skin—peach or orange counteracts blue tones, while pink addresses yellow undertones and sallowness.*

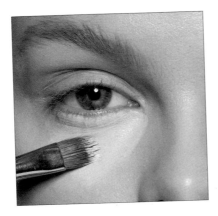

concealer

With the many colors and consistencies of concealer available, you can usually hide anything from a simple blemish to dark under-eye circles, scarring, birthmarks, and even tattoos. Today's concealers can be sheer, lightweight, and natural, but they can flatten raised spots and mask discoloration when applied in the right way.

cream concealer This gives full coverage and is very easy to apply; it works well underneath the eyes and on older skin.

stick concealer This has a thicker consistency and can be a little drying but is good for blemishes and easy to apply directly on the area that needs it.

liquid Usually in the form of a pen or wand, this multipurpose concealer is easy to blend but gives quite light coverage.

pencils Ideal for touch-ups, these give medium coverage.

mineral powder concealer A great option for sensitive skin, it is easy to apply and gives good coverage for dark circles.

highlighters Containing light-reflective particles, these sheer products are good for brightening an area and lightening dark circles but they don't give much coverage.

camouflage These heavy-duty concealers are the ones to use for covering birthmarks, scars, and tattoos.

dark circles

Peachy pink color corrector will counteract the bruised appearance of the skin underneath tired eyes and have a brightening effect. If you need to use a concealer as well, choose a creamy consistency that isn't too heavy, as you don't want a cakey effect. Press it into the skin gently so you don't rub off the color corrector underneath.

broken capillaries

These fine, spidery thread veins sometimes appear across the cheeks and around the nose. They are often hereditary but can also be caused by extremes of temperature. Creamy foundation or light foundation and concealer could be enough to cover them, but you may need a touch of yellow or green color corrector too.

scars

Exfoliate the area very gently and then moisturize it well to ensure the surface is clean and as smooth as possible. If the scar is red or purple, use green or peach color correctors to address this. Then apply a highly pigmented camouflage product, which has a thicker consistency for maximum coverage. Set with loose powder or a setting spray.

spots

Keep the area clean and use an antibacterial treatment to help dry out the spot and reduce inflammation; try not to touch it. Your skincare routine is important—choose products that are formulated to balance spot-prone skin. Address redness with yellow or green color corrector and then use an oil-free concealer to cover it.

rosacea

Yellow or green color corrector, depending on your skin tone, will help to neutralize the redness in your cheeks. The sun aggravates the condition, so always wear sunscreen. Choose oil-free concealer and foundation that give sufficient coverage—anything sheer won't work. Avoid blush and any tones that will accentuate your natural redness.

age spots

Hyperpigmentation is caused by an increased production of melanin in the skin, which is caused by UV rays through overexposure to the sun. Orange and violet color correctors can be used to help neutralize age spots. Camouflage concealers and heavier cream foundations let you build coverage without giving a cakey finish.

Foundation

As its name suggests, foundation is a skin-colored make-up base that is applied to the face to help even out skin tone, cover blemishes, and create a smooth complexion. It comes in many formats, from powders, liquids, and creams to gels, mousses, and sprays. Coverage varies from light to heavy, and finishes may be sheer, dewy, creamy, or matte. Many "smart" foundations incorporate sunscreen, illuminators, hydrators, moisturizers, mattifiers, or anti-aging ingredients. Choose one that is suitable for your skin type, matches your skin color, and gives you the amount of coverage you require.

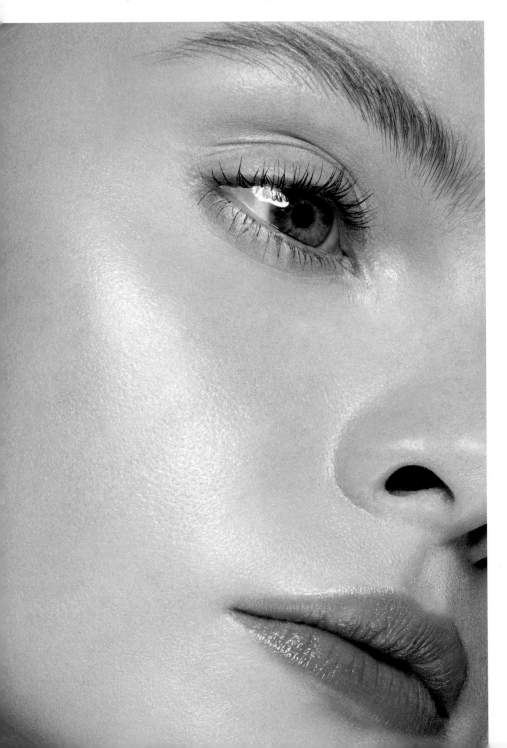

tinted moisturizer ←

This gives a very light, sheer coverage that allows the natural skin to show through, so it's ideal for people who already have good skin and want a very "bare" make-up look. It evens out the skin tone in a natural way and gives a fresh, dewy finish. The moisturizing formulas usually contain sunscreen and often other skincare, anti-aging, or illuminating ingredients. In general, it suits normal or dry skin; I wouldn't use it on oily or sensitive skin.

liquid →

One of the most popular types of foundation, this may be oil-based, water-based, or waterproof, lightweight or heavier in consistency. People often think liquid foundation is really light and sheer, but it's very easy to layer and can be built up to achieve good coverage. Liquid foundation is hydrating and moisturizing, making it good for most skin types. Many also incorporate sunscreen, illuminators, and active skincare ingredients. You will usually need to set it with powder.

bb/cc creams

Blemish Balm and Color Corrector creams have taken the make-up world by storm. These multitaskers combine skincare and perfecting properties, acting as an all-in-one moisturizer, serum, primer, foundation, and concealer/color corrector. They have the consistency of tinted moisturizer but vary enormously in the level of coverage they provide.

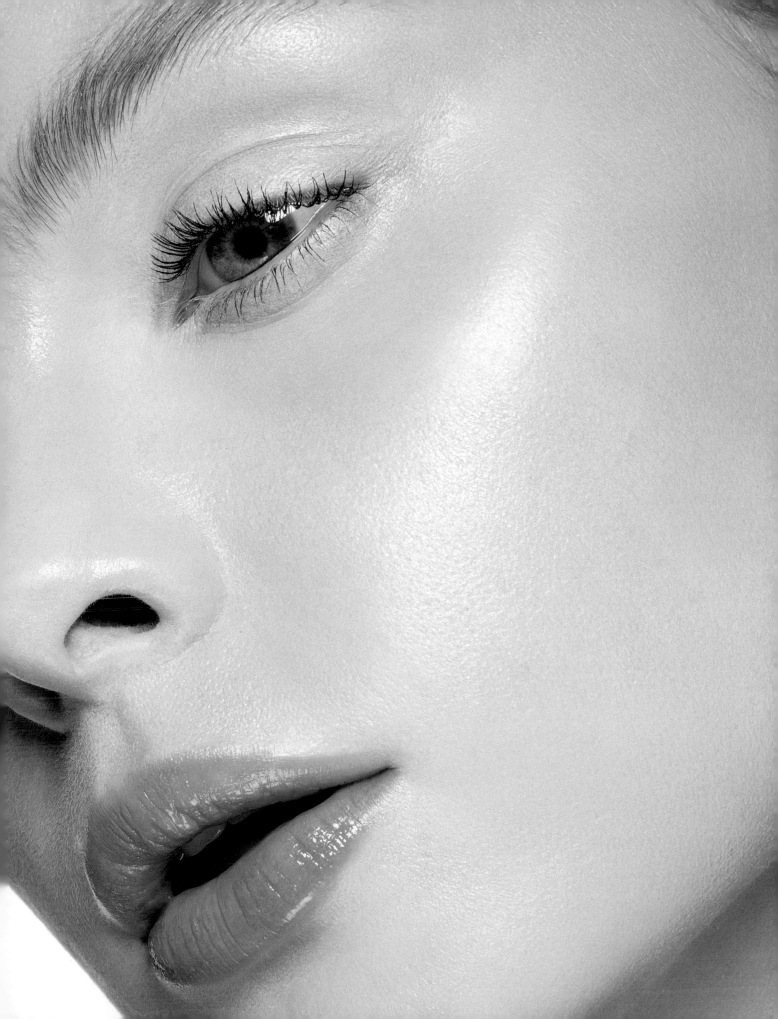

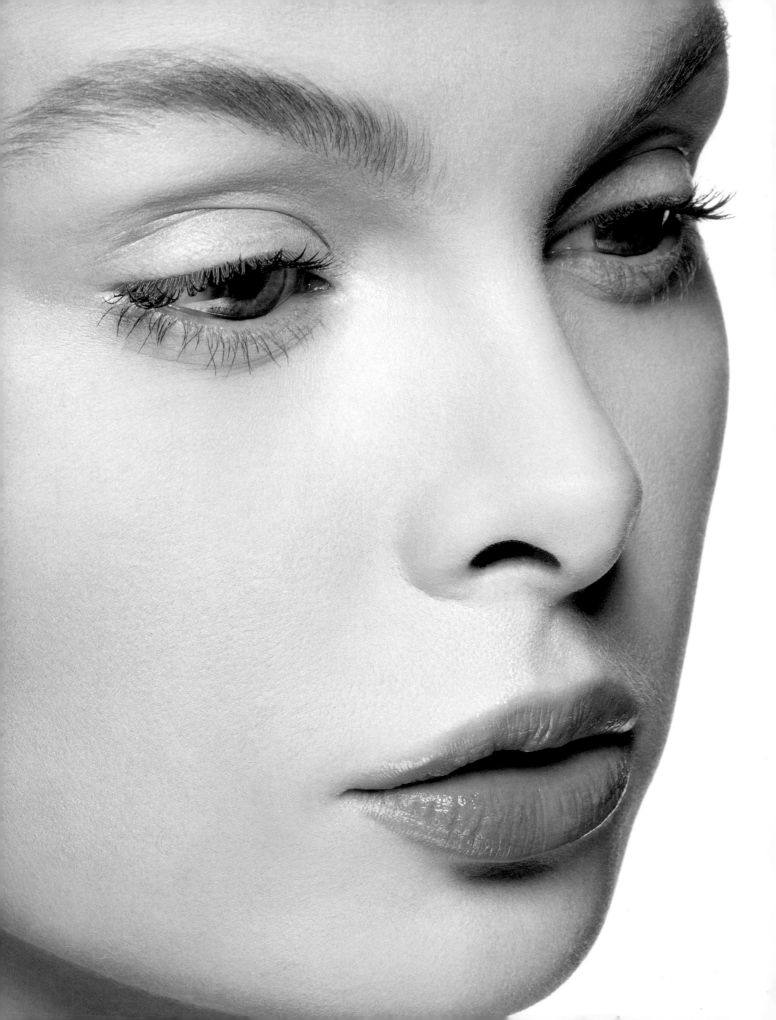

powder/mineral ←

This foundation-and-powder-in-one comes pressed in a compact or as loose powder in shades to suit all skin tones. It's portable, convenient, and easy to apply for light to medium coverage. Be careful when you build it up, as it can change the skin tone and look dirty and heavy. Powder foundation cancels out shine on oily skin while letting it breathe, but is not suitable for dry, flaky skin. It's great for setting make-up and can be combined with other foundations—I often apply it over liquid or cream foundation to give extra coverage where needed. If you have oily skin, blot the face with a tissue before application to prevent patchiness. Mineral foundation is healing and protects the skin from UV rays, giving medium to full coverage. It doesn't clog the pores and is often anti-inflammatory for skin conditions such as rosacea, but some people find it drying. Always use a powder blush on top of powder foundation.

cream/stick →

This thick, creamy formulation comes in a compact or as a stick and gives an even finish with medium to full coverage—a stick gives the heaviest coverage. It's great for normal, dry, or older skin but can be too rich for oily skin. It's easy to apply and is long-lasting and moisturizing. Cream-to-powder foundation goes on like cream but dries to a powdery finish. This is time- and money-saving, and a great option for oily skin.

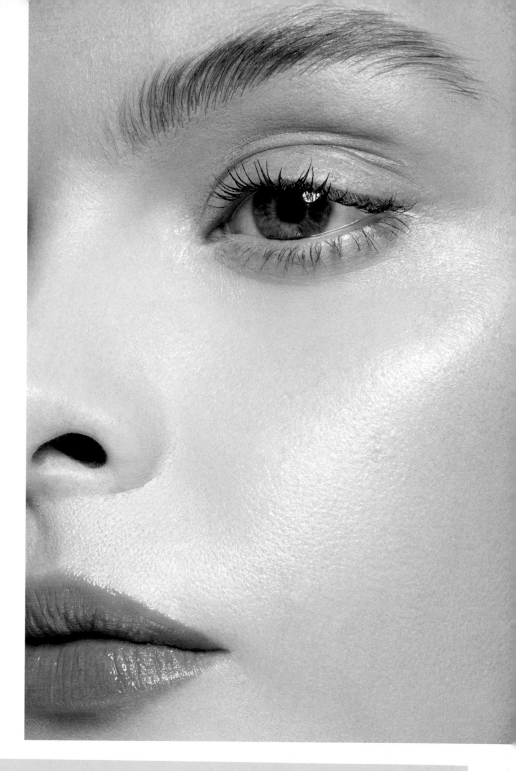

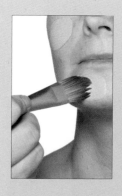
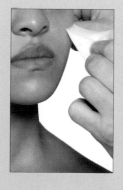

application

I generally apply liquid formulations—primer, tinted moisturizer, BB/CC cream, or liquid foundation—with a tapered, angled, synthetic foundation brush, wedge-shaped sponge, or egg-shaped beauty blender, but you can use your fingertips if you prefer. Cream foundation can be applied with a flat-topped synthetic brush, sponge, or beauty blender; if you're contouring, use a buffing brush to connect the shades. There is a wide choice of sizes and shapes of contour brushes, cut to fit the cheekbone or nose, for example, to make application easier. Powder foundation should be polished into the skin with a soft brush, such as a fat, flat-topped kabuki brush.

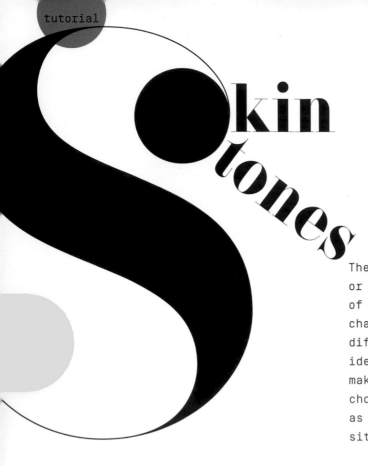

Skin tones

The color of human skin varies from the palest creamy or pinkish white to the darkest brown. The perception of which tone within this range is desirable has changed continually throughout the years and in different cultures. It's necessary to be able to identify your skin tone in order to choose the correct make-up. This is especially important when it comes to choosing foundation, as you want it to look as natural as possible and disappear into your skin rather than sit on the surface like a mask.

The quantity and type of melanin, a brown or black pigment produced by skin cells called melanocytes, determine how dark the skin will be. In lighter skin, which has less melanin, the color of the connective tissue under the skin's dermis (a bluish white) and the hemoglobin inside the red blood cells (a bluish red or red, depending on whether it is deoxygenated or oxygenated) also comes into play. This is why skin that is very pale and almost translucent often has a bluish undertone and why pale people often flush noticeably as blood rushes to the surface of the skin.

Melanin protects the skin from burning UV rays and is produced in response to sun exposure, resulting in a "tan." Although skin tone is a genetic predisposition, a number of factors can affect it, such as exposure to the sun, aging (which can lead to hyperpigmentation—brown "liver spots" on paler skin and ashy patches on darker skin), hormonal changes (skin darkens during puberty, for example), and conditions such as rosacea and acne.

skin tone test

Skin tones are classified as being warm, cool, or neutral. A quick test is to look at the veins on the underside of your wrist: if the veins look greenish, your skin tone is warm; if they appear pink or blush-colored, your skin tone is cool; if you are a mixture, you have a neutral or balanced skin tone. There's also the so-called "jewelry test:" if gold jewelry looks best against your skin, your skin tone is probably warm; if platinum and silver suit you better, your skin tone is likely to be cool. However, fashion and personal preference are likely to influence your choices. Below are some generalizations:

warm Eyes are often brown, hazel, or green; hair is likely to be black, brown, red, or blonde; skin has yellow, peach, or olive undertones.

cool Eyes are probably blue, green, or brown; hair is usually blonde, brown, or black; skin has blue or pink undertones.

neutral Eyes and hair can be any color; skin is a balanced mix of pink and blue undertones and it is hard to specify just one.

light/porcelain

Very pale skin usually goes hand in hand with blonde or dark hair and has pink undertones. It is often quite transparent and burns easily, so sunscreen is essential. There is usually not as much choice in the very light shades of foundation, but it's important to get it right so it doesn't look fake. Any texture will work, but tinted moisturizer might be too sheer because the skin is so transparent. Stick to subtle blushes that don't contain too much pigment or they will look too strong.

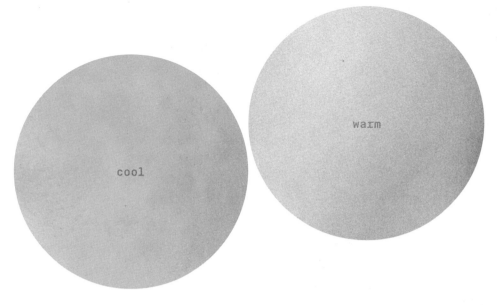

cool

warm

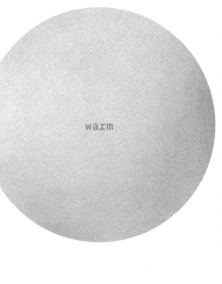

warm

cool

fair

Although it tends to be more yellow-based than light skin, fair skin can still have predominantly pink undertones. It can often look quite pale in the winter but have more color in the summer, and it is prone to burning in the sun but will then tan. A foundation that is too pale will make you look like a ghost, so it's a good idea to have two shades that you can blend together to get a perfect match all year. Peach or apricot blushes and champagne highlighters will suit you.

medium

This type of skin, which includes those of Latino, Mediterranean, and Asian heritage, generally tans easily in the sun and often goes with dark hair and either dark or blue eyes. There's a wide range of foundation shades to choose from, and having two shades can help you achieve a perfect match through the seasons. Color looks great on your skin, so you can choose more highly pigmented blushes, but avoid anything too light or frosted, as it will look ashy.

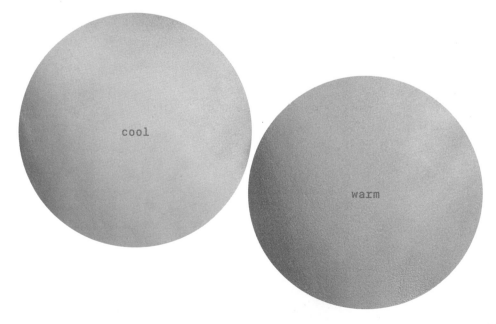

cool

warm

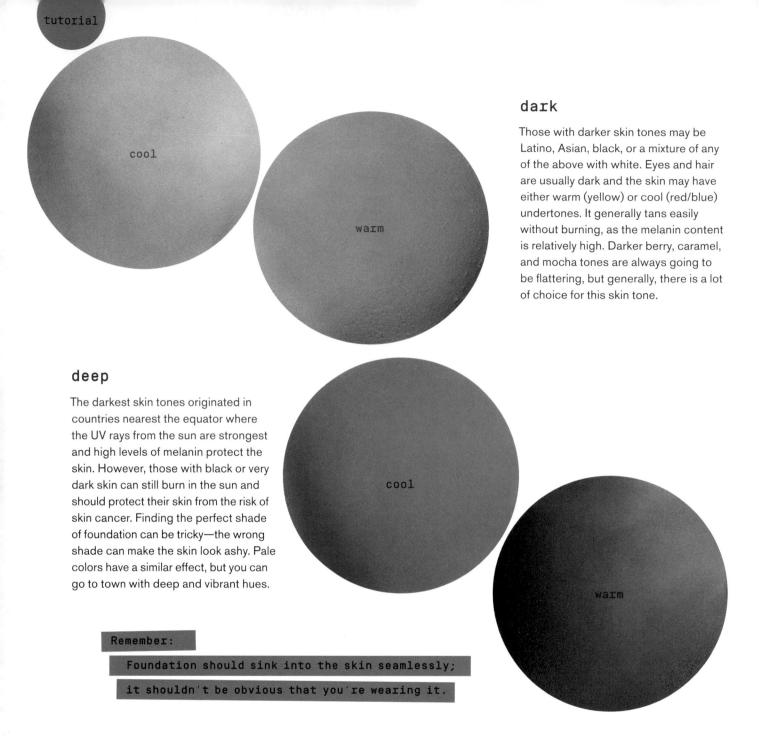

dark

Those with darker skin tones may be Latino, Asian, black, or a mixture of any of the above with white. Eyes and hair are usually dark and the skin may have either warm (yellow) or cool (red/blue) undertones. It generally tans easily without burning, as the melanin content is relatively high. Darker berry, caramel, and mocha tones are always going to be flattering, but generally, there is a lot of choice for this skin tone.

deep

The darkest skin tones originated in countries nearest the equator where the UV rays from the sun are strongest and high levels of melanin protect the skin. However, those with black or very dark skin can still burn in the sun and should protect their skin from the risk of skin cancer. Finding the perfect shade of foundation can be tricky—the wrong shade can make the skin look ashy. Pale colors have a similar effect, but you can go to town with deep and vibrant hues.

Remember:

Foundation should sink into the skin seamlessly; it shouldn't be obvious that you're wearing it.

color match

When looking for a foundation, you need to try to match your underlying skin tone; the foundation will then neutralize the overtones in your skin to even it out. When I'm choosing foundation for someone, I initially pick three or four shades by eye that I think will work on them. It's important to look at the skin in daylight, as artificial light casts its own color onto the skin and won't give you a true match. I'll then apply a little of each one—whether it's a liquid, cream, or powde—to the jawline with my finger, a sponge, or brush. If you can see the foundation and the color is obviously

lighter or darker than the skin, then it's the wrong color. If it disappears and melts into the skin, then it's the right color. Take it a little way down onto the neck to double-check. You can't do this on your hand or arm, as the skin there has a different texture and tone from the skin on your face and won't give you an accurate match. Sometimes you can get the color match right straightaway—there's such a wide range of foundations out there that there's something for everyone. If not, you may have to customize by blending colors together—as a make-up artist, I do this quite often.

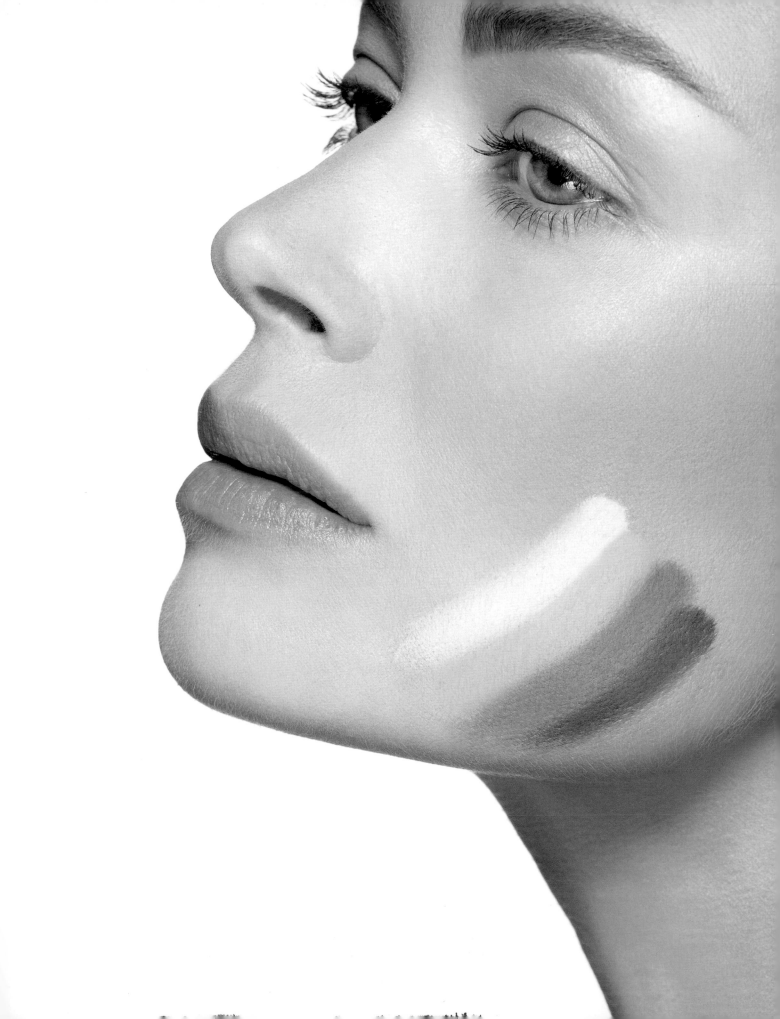

Barely there

Everyone wants naturally flawless skin, and this look is all about achieving a glowing complexion using soft, nude colors that gently enhance the skin tone.

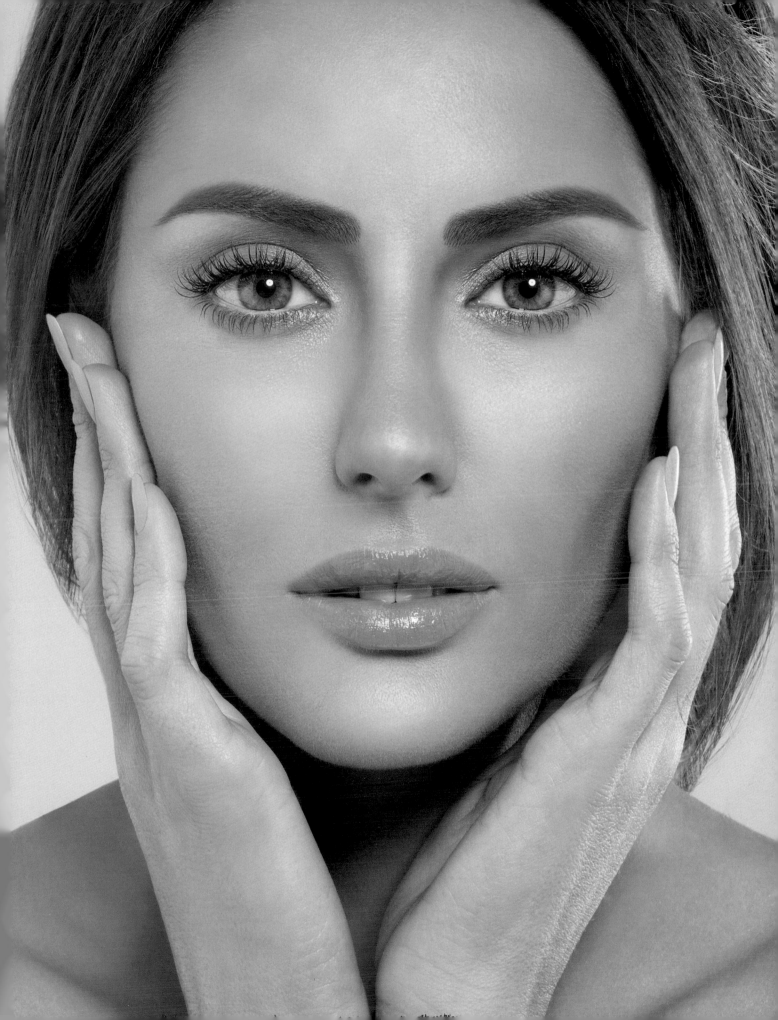

Barely There Transformation

Everyone would like to wake up in the morning and look amazing, but few people feel confident enough to go out with no make-up on at all. Inner health is a key factor and there are many small lifestyle changes you can make that will help to improve the appearance of your skin [see pages 22-5], but expertly applied make-up will instantly brighten any complexion. The aim of this understated look is to achieve perfect, luminous skin using natural tones and textures, but to seem as though you are wearing little or no make-up. With the focus on radiant skin that exudes health and youth, and eyes and lips accentuated in a simple,

fabulous way, it doesn't take long to do and will give you the confidence to step out into the world. Our model [previous spread] has fair skin, so I used a mix of warm, apricot-based neutrals and moisturizing tinted lip balm for a natural, daytime look. For Chloe's transformation, I concentrated on color-correcting and evening out the skin tone to achieve a perfect complexion. Selecting the correct foundation is key to creating a flawless finish—darker skin can look sallow or "ashy" if the tone isn't right, so don't be afraid to mix shades together to create a perfect match.

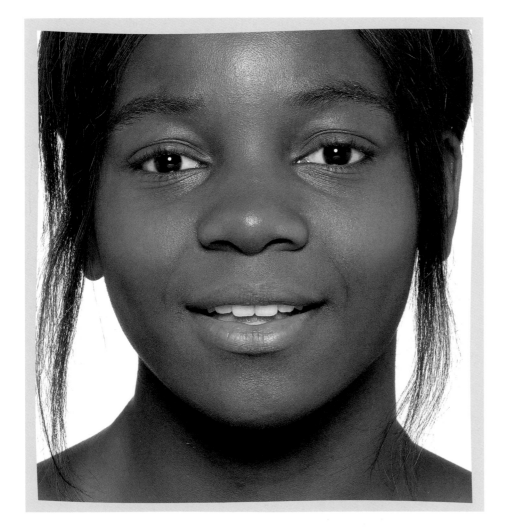

Chloe is 21 so her skin has a natural, youthful freshness, but no one has perfect skin or a completely even skin tone and she often finds it difficult to color-match products to her skin. I wanted to show that nude shades with the same undertones as your skin will always look flattering, whatever your age or coloring.

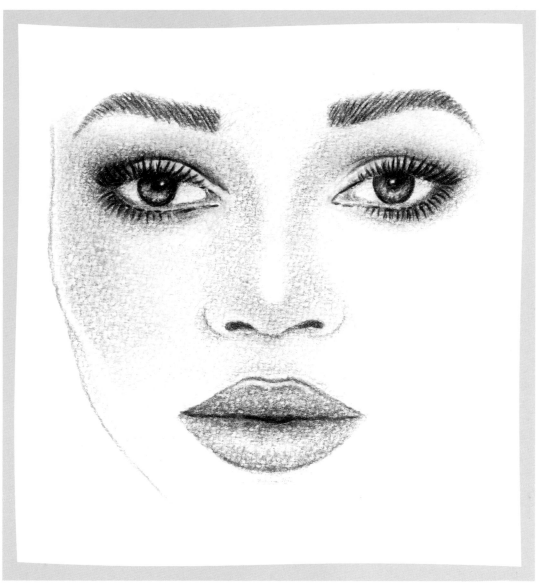

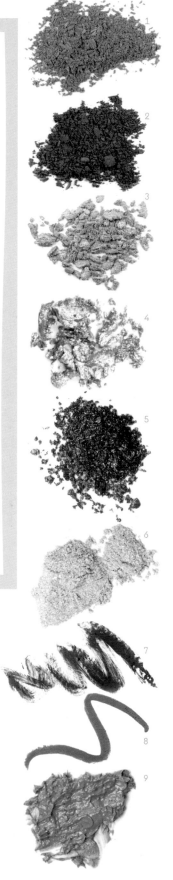

face

Hydrating primer.
Lightweight moisturizing,
illuminating liquid foundation
to match the skin tone.
Darker and lighter shades
of the same foundation
for contouring.
Two tones of powder to
set the contouring.
Warm apricot and brown
powder blushes (1 and 2).
Champagne-colored
highlighter (3).

eyes

Mid-brown matte
brow powder.
Champagne-colored
eyeshadow with a slight
shimmer (4).
Chocolate-brown eyeshadow
with a slight shimmer (5).
Vanilla shimmer pigment (6).
Black gel eyeliner (7).
Black mascara.

lips

Soft brown lip liner (8).
Creamy, warm caramel-
brown lipstick (9).
Clear lip gloss.

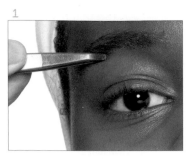

■face

1 First, I prepared her face by cleansing, toning, and moisturizing (see pages 28–9). Then I tweezed away any stray hairs from underneath her eyebrows, still keeping them very natural but creating a nice, clean arch.

2 Chloe has combination skin so I used a hydrating primer all over her face, including her eyelids, for a natural glow. I then applied a lightweight, moisturizing, illuminating liquid foundation, using a make-up sponge for a smooth finish. To even out her skin tone and brighten the eye area, I used two different shades of the same foundation—one that was about two shades lighter around the eyes, along the top of the cheekbones, on the tip of the chin, the bridge of the nose, and the center of the forehead, and one that matched her skin tone to create shadow under the jawline, at the temples, down the sides of the nose, and under the cheekbones. You could use concealer instead of a lighter foundation, but it's usually a heavier consistency and can settle into fine lines, which can be aging.

3 I blended the foundations into her skin well with a brush. This is a simple way to contour the face for a natural result.

4 Using a large, angled, natural-bristle brush, I set the foundation using two tones of powder, blending it well, as before, for a flawless finish. If you want a lighter finish, just use a dusting of translucent powder to set the foundation.

5 To give her nose a slimmer appearance, I applied a contouring powder two shades darker than her skin tone down both sides and under the base of the nose to lift it up a little, using a small brush for precision. Then I applied a lighter shade along the bridge and on the tip to draw the eye.

6–7 To bring a luminous glow to the skin, I used a blend of warm brown and apricot powder blush and champagne-colored highlighter. Following the contour that I'd made on her cheeks, I applied a blend of the brown and apricot tones in the mid-section, between the light and dark, starting near the ear and working down. Then I added a touch to the apples of the cheeks. The key is to make sure you don't take the blush too close to the mouth, so lift the brush off the skin when you reach the apple and then add a little color to the apple itself. I then brushed highlighter along the top of the cheekbones, the bridge of the nose, the center of the chin, forehead, and brow bones. This combination of soft, warm tones really brings life and color to her face.

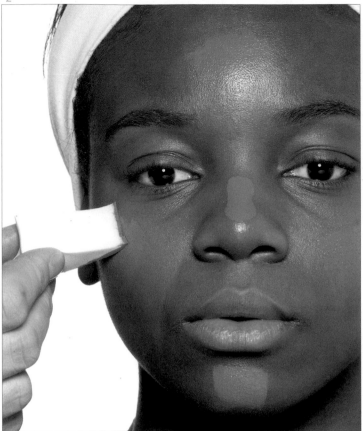

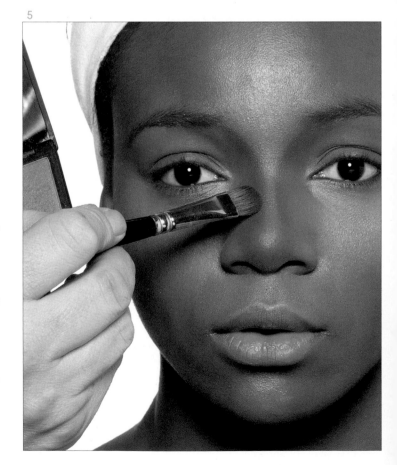

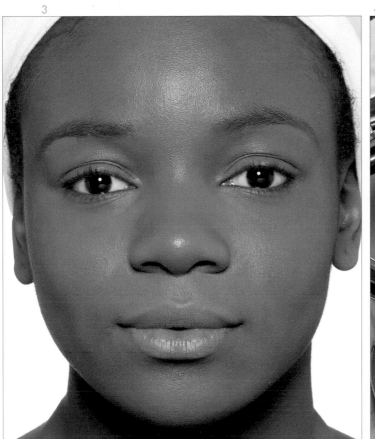

3

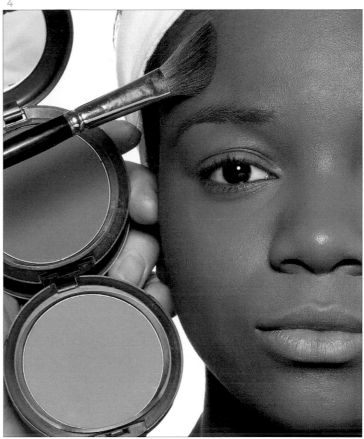

4

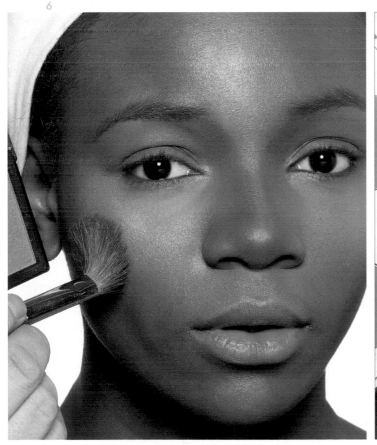

6

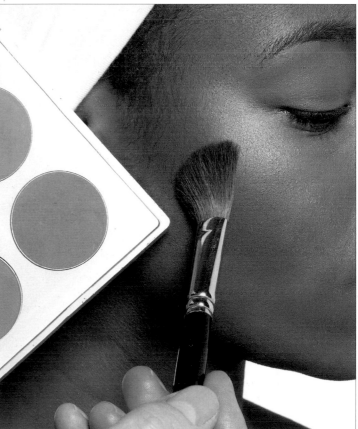

7

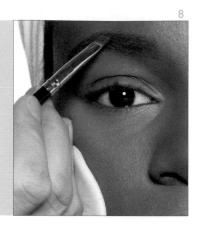

If I need to
steady my hand,
I place a clean
powder puff
between my hand
and the cheek so
I don't smudge
the make-up.

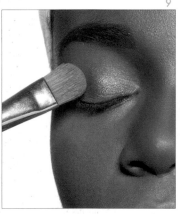

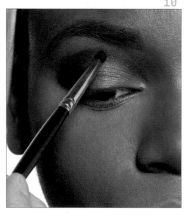

▪eyes

8 I filled in the eyebrows using a mid-brown matte brow powder and a soft angled brush for a precise finish. This resulted in a more defined arch with a fuller shape that still looked very soft and natural.

9 For the eyes, I chose a champagne-colored eyeshadow with a slight shimmer and applied it all over the eyelid, blending it upward and outward toward the brow bone to create a soft wash. Shimmer eyeshadow has a brightening effect and is very easy to blend.

10 Using a chocolate-brown eyeshadow with a slight shimmer and a small round pencil brush, I cut out a soft crease just above the natural socket line to give the impression of a bigger, wider eye. I started at the outer edge of the eye, swept the darker shade into the crease, and then blended it with the lighter color.

11 Then I swept the same brown eyeshadow under the lower lash line, starting at the outer corner of the eye, where the color is deeper, and sweeping it lightly toward the inner corner.

12 I blended the colors really well and then added an accent of vanilla shimmer pigment to the beginning of the eye to really open it up.

13 I defined the upper and lower lash lines with a black gel liner and a small angled brush. (You could use a soft pencil liner if you find that easier.) I then used a small round pencil brush to smudge and soften the lower line.

14 I curled the upper lashes from roots to tips and then applied black mascara to the top and bottom lashes to create volume but still keep the look natural.

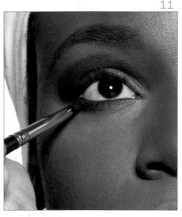

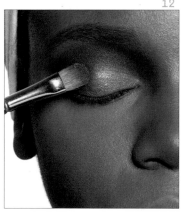

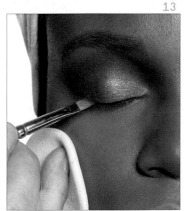

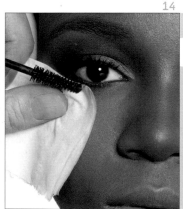

Tip When applying mascara, hold
a tissue under the lower
lashes, right up to the roots.
When you put the wand onto the
lower lashes and wiggle it
through them, the tissue will
protect the skin underneath.

■ lips

15 Chloe's bottom lip is slightly fuller than her top lip, so I wanted to even out the shape a little. I used a soft brown lip liner and drew the outline just a fraction outside the upper lip line and a fraction inside the lower lip line.

16 So there are no hard lines on the finished look, I blended this a little way into the lips with a lip brush and then applied a creamy, warm, caramel-brown lipstick on top, blending it together well.

17 To finish, I added a touch of clear gloss to the center of the bottom lip. For a daytime look, you don't need to use the gloss and you could choose a natural tinted lip balm or sheer lipstick for a lighter look.

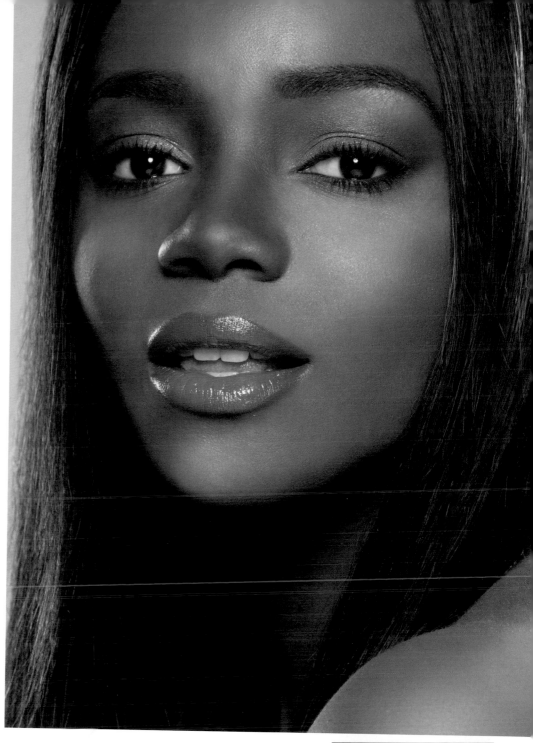

15

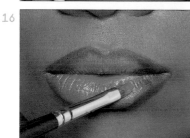

16

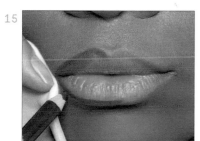

17

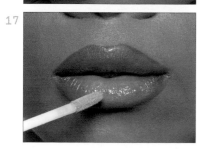

"This make-up is very glamorous and sophisticated but still quite subtle and understated. The combination of neutral colors Gary chose really suited my skin tone and I love how flawless and polished my skin looks."

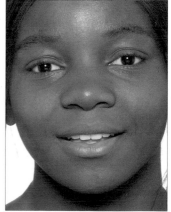

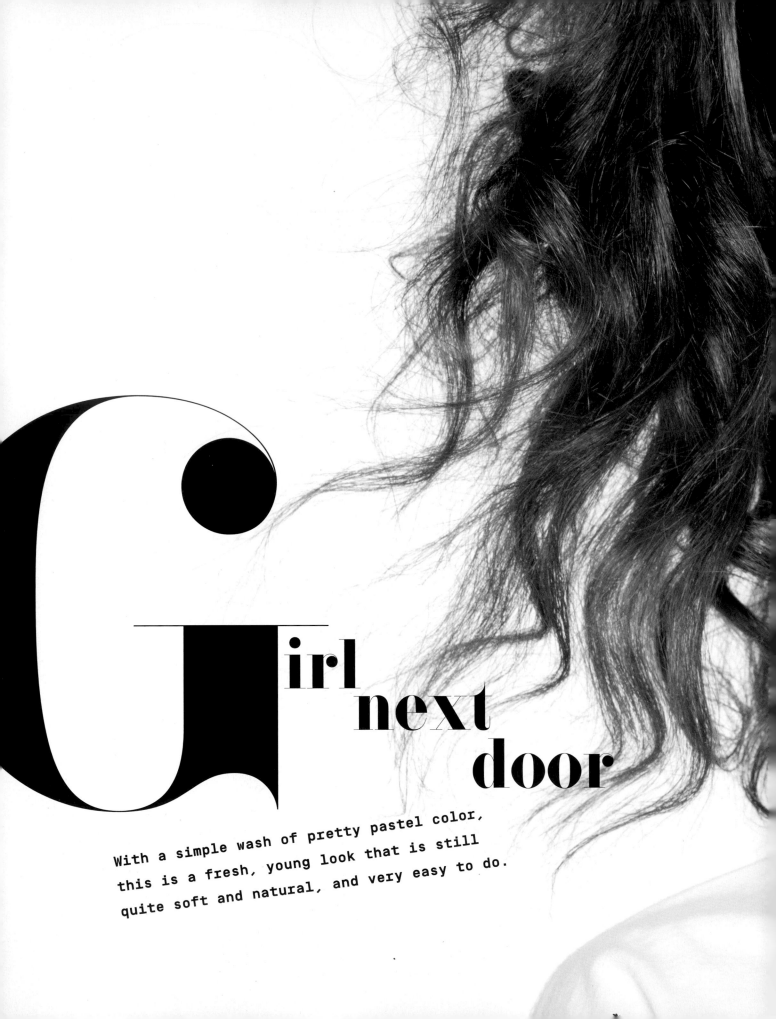

Girl next door

With a simple wash of pretty pastel color, this is a fresh, young look that is still quite soft and natural, and very easy to do.

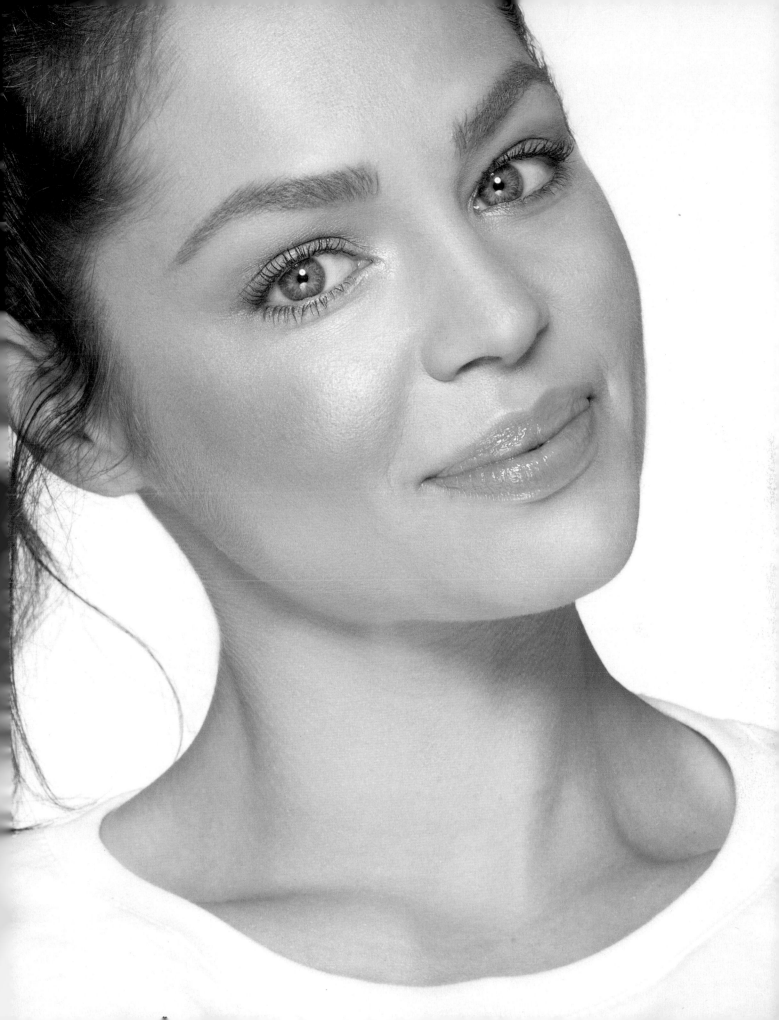

Girl Next Door Transformation

The Girl Next Door is an innocent, fresh-faced look that is as sweet and wholesome as apple pie—there is nothing extreme or edgy about this make-up. It's all about natural, clear skin with a youthful glow and a healthy flush to the cheeks. A great tip for finding the perfect shade of blush is to pinch your cheeks and match the color to the natural pigment in your skin. This look is perfect for young girls who are just discovering make-up, as the light coverage lets the skin's radiance shine through, while the wash of pretty pastel on the lids gives you the chance to play around with different tones and textures. Experiment with mouthwatering pastels in sugared-almond shades or play it safe with soft neutrals. Colorwashes are very versatile and easy to apply; you can use either a shimmer powder, which is easy to blend, or a cream finish. Cream textures stay in place better on tight, young skin, but are not as forgiving on the eyes, as they tend to sink into creases. On our model [previous spread] I used a cream eyeshadow in petal-pink, a tinted lip balm in the same tone, and a shimmer-brick blush for added glow. For the transformation on Georgina, I chose a lilac powder eyeshadow with a slight shimmer to bring out the green of her eyes.

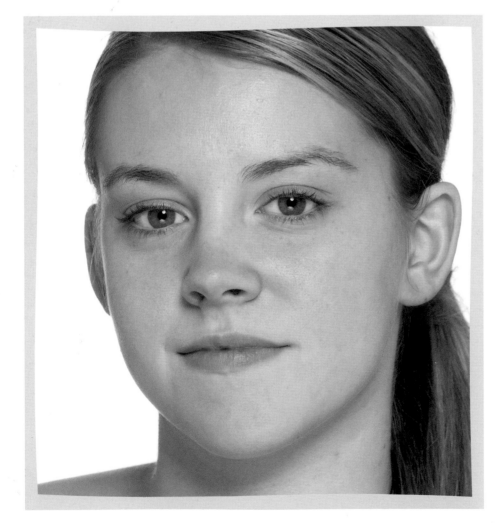

Georgina is 18 and has just started to experiment with make-up, so I wanted to show her an easy look that would bring out the freshness of her skin and complement her youthful glow. She's a fun girl and this look sums up her personality beautifully.

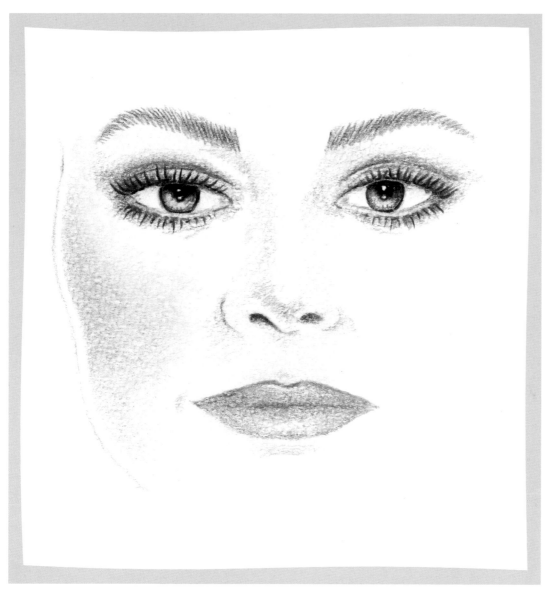

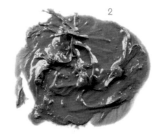

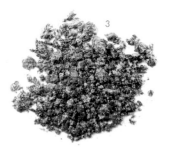

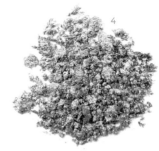

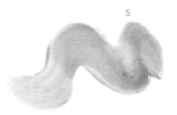

face
Oil-free primer.
Sheer tinted moisturizer
to match the skin tone.
Concealer.
Cream highlighter (1).
Bright rose-pink cream
blush (2).
Translucent powder.

eyes
Ash-blonde matte
brow powder.
Pastel lilac eyeshadow with
a slight shimmer (3).
Lighter lilac shimmery pigment
eyeshadow (4).
Dark brown/black mascara.

lips
Fresh pink lip gloss (5).

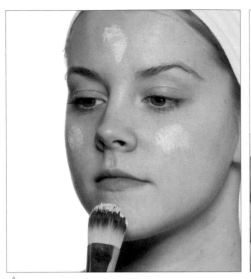

1

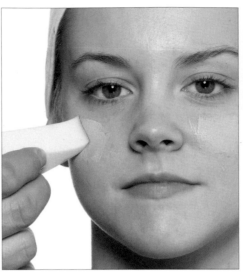

2

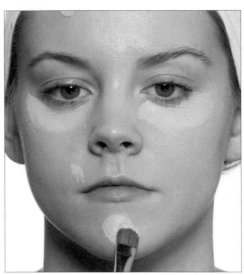

3

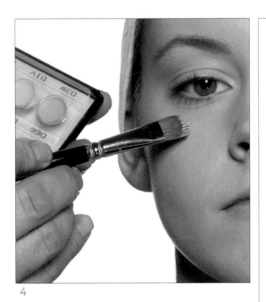

4

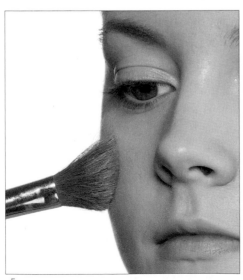

5

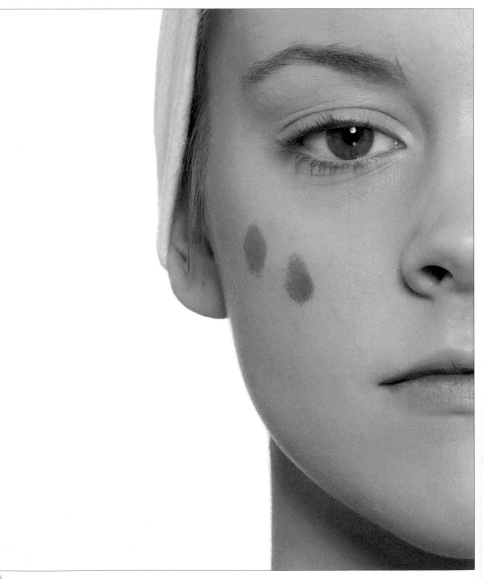

6

This is an ideal look for using a time-saving multipurpose product. Choose a cream or stick in pink, peach, coral, or caramel tones and use it on the eyes, cheeks, and lips.

Tips

» Colorwashes look great in cream eyeshadow, which you can apply with a brush or your finger.

» Choose a lip gloss in a shade that works with the eyeshadow color and complements your skin tone.

» If you prefer less shiny lips, blot the colored gloss with a tissue or use a lipstick with a satin finish.

▪face

1 Georgina has typical teenage skin—slightly on the oily side with a few little blemishes— so after prepping her face (see pages 28–9), I applied an oil-free primer to create a good, even base.

2 I then applied quite a sheer tinted moisturizer to the T-zone and blended it outward with a sponge. Tinted moisturizer works well on oily complexions and is ideal for young skin, as it evens out skin tones without covering freckles, creating a fresh, natural finish with only light coverage.

3 I brushed a little concealer onto any areas that needed extra help—to cover a few small blemishes and to brighten the under-eye area—and blended it into the foundation.

4 To add a fresh glow to her skin, I blended a cream highlighter along the top of the cheekbones, down the bridge of the nose, and in the center of the chin.

5 I then powdered her face with a very light dusting of translucent powder to set the base and take away any unwanted shine.

6–7 For a natural, youthful flush, I dotted some bright rose-pink cream blush onto the mid-section of her cheeks and blended it well using a brush (you could use your fingertips for this if you find it easier), keeping the color on the apples of the cheeks.

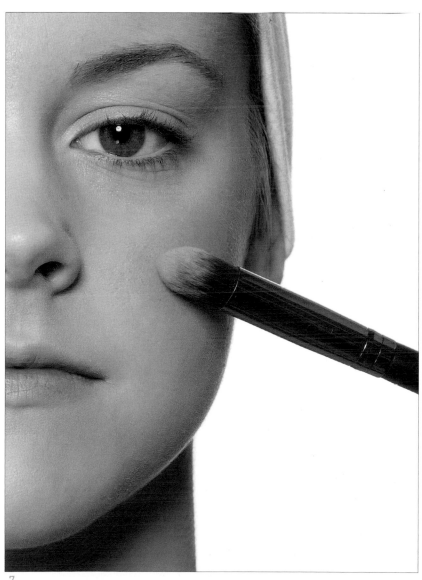

7

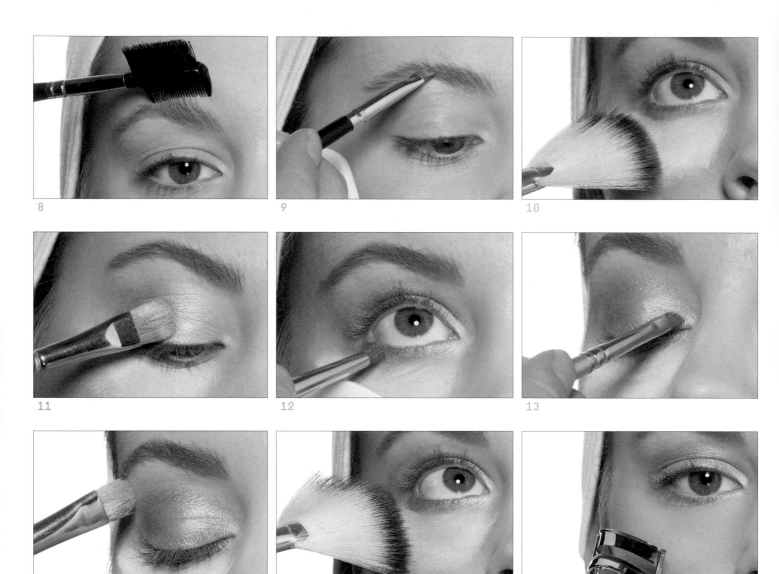

eyes

8 Having tweezed away any stray hairs, I brushed the eyebrows up.

9 Then I filled in any areas that needed it using an ash-blonde brow powder to create a very natural, soft arch.

10 To protect the make-up on the face, I applied a thin layer of translucent powder beneath the eyes—if any eyeshadow drops onto the face, it can be brushed away when the eye is finished.

11 Using a medium-sized eyeshadow brush, I applied a wash of pastel lilac

eyeshadow with a slight shimmer over the whole lid and blended it out with a soft blending brush.

12 Starting at the outer corner, I then swept the same color underneath the eye, close to the lash line, and blended it toward the center with a soft round pencil brush.

13 Using a small angled brush for precision, I added a shimmery pigment eyeshadow in a lighter shade of lilac around the tear duct and under the eye at the inner corner to brighten the area and make the eyes look more awake.

14 With a soft brush, I blended the outer edges so the colorwash faded softly into the brow bone.

15 Having finished the eyeshadow, I swept away the powder underneath the eyes with a fan brush, starting at the beginning of the eye and sweeping it outward with a couple of swift strokes, to leave clear skin underneath.

16 I curled the upper lashes and applied dark brown mascara to the top and bottom lashes; you could use black mascara, but Georgina is blonde and I didn't want to overpower the look.

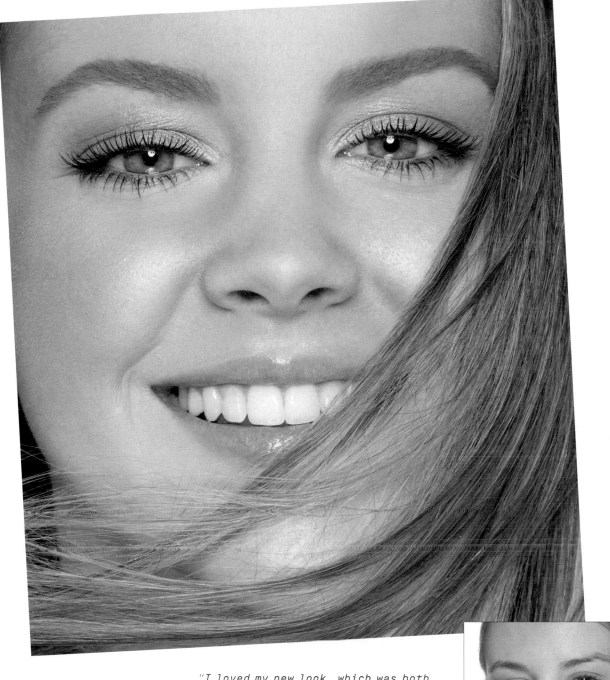

"I loved my new look, which was both fun and accessible. My boyfriend hates me wearing make-up but loved how natural I looked and that I still looked like me."

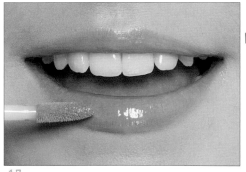

■lips

17 To keep the lips looking as natural as possible, I didn't line them with a pencil but just chose a fresh, pink gloss for a simple, shiny finish. If you prefer, you can matte it down with a tissue or use a lipstick with a satin finish. Choose a fresh pink that works with the eyes and complements your skin.

17

Contour

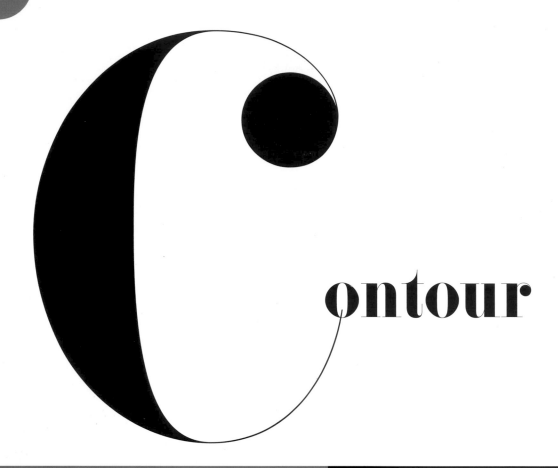

Being able to contour your face is one of the most useful make-up skills you can master. Contouring is the art of using light and dark to enhance certain features and play down others. It can be used to sculpt cheekbones, chisel jaws, hide double chins, slim down wide noses, and lower high foreheads. This simple art of illusion works on the principle that dark colors make things recede and light colors bring them forward. You can either use a contouring kit or choose a creamy foundation two to three shades darker than your natural skin tone and another two to three shades lighter. Make sure all the colors have the same undertone that works with your skin tone. You can use powder if you prefer: the dark shade must be matte but the lighter shade can have a slight sheen to reflect the light. I sometimes use powders as well as foundation, both to set the contouring and to make it more dramatic. The general principles are shown on pages 58-9; see how to contour different face shapes on pages 60-1.

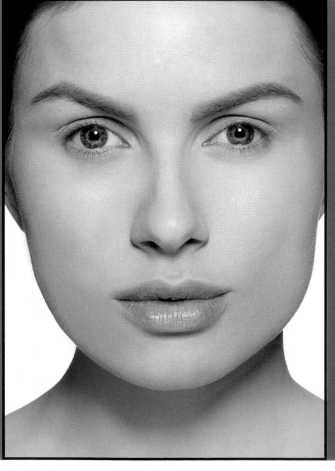

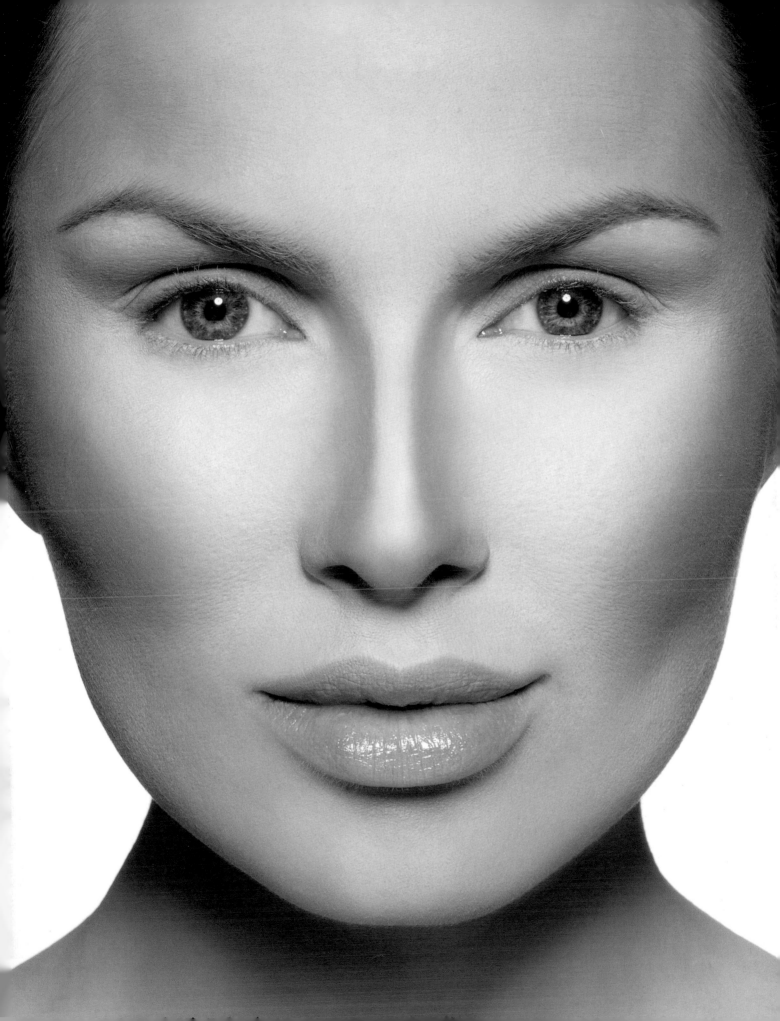

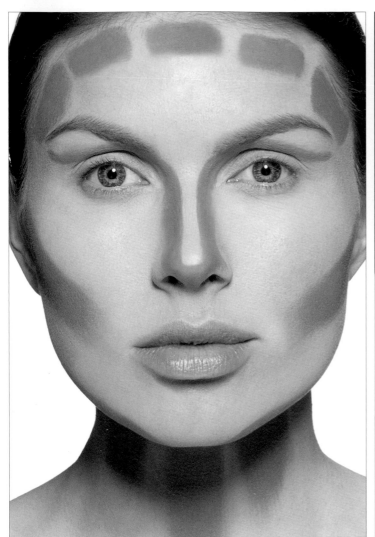

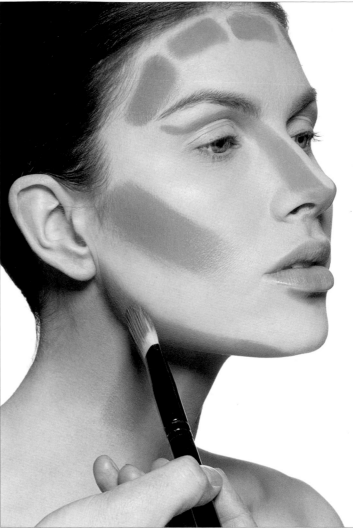

create shadow

Prepare your face as usual—moisturize, prime, and tidy your brows—and then apply a light liquid foundation, tinted moisturizer, or BB cream.

Start with the cutting out. I used a medium-sized, flat contouring brush but there are lots of brushes to choose from. Apply the darker color under and in line with your cheekbones, starting at the hairline and pushing the color into the center of the face in a single sweep. Don't take the color too far in, and create softness in the center of the face.

Take the color from the bottom of your ear along your jawline, making sure it is even on both sides. This helps to create definition and soften a heavy jaw.

Sweep the darker color under your chin and down your neck. This helps to lift the jaw, disguising a double chin and creating a more youthful appearance.

To soften the temples and minimize a high or wide forehead, apply the dark color from the end of the eyebrows all the way around the hairline.

Use a slightly smaller brush to contour the nose, mouth, and eyes. To slim your nose, start at the top and apply the dark shade down both sides with a steady hand, taking the color slightly onto the top of the nose and under its tip.

Apply a dab of dark color underneath the lower lip in the center of the mouth. This pushes the area back, making the lips appear to come forward and seem fuller.

Define the socket line to create a crease to give the eyes depth.

Remember:

To enhance and bring forward, add light;

to play down and push back, add dark.

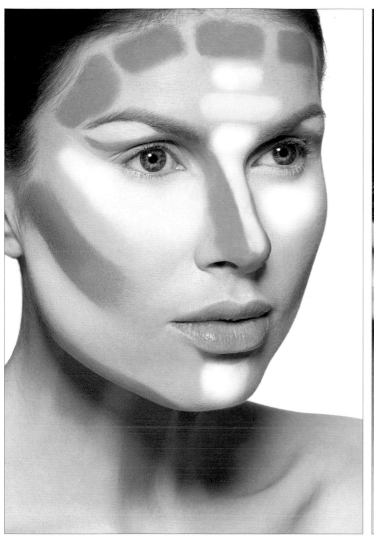

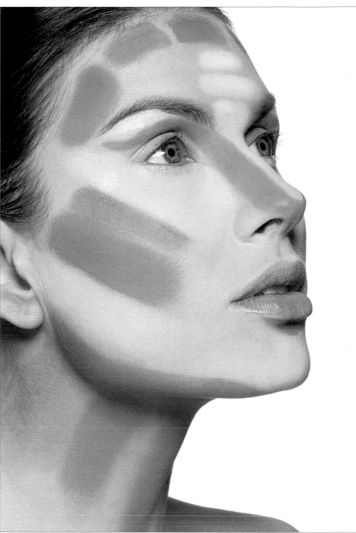

create light

Then apply the light color to the areas that you want to add light to and draw the eye toward. Stand in good natural light and look in a mirror. The parts of your face on which light falls naturally are the areas to highlight.

Using a clean, medium-sized, flat contouring brush (or brush of your choice), apply the lighter color underneath the eyes to minimize any dark shadows, flatten out the area, and bring it forward. Draw a triangle shape following the contour of the eye socket, sweeping up to the outer corner and stopping in line with the end of your eyebrows.

Sweep the lighter color along your lower face from your hairline toward your chin between the two areas of darker color.

Using a clean, smaller flat brush, apply the lighter color to the center of your chin and above your upper lip.

Apply the lighter color to the middle of your forehead and take it down the very center of your nose.

blush

Draw pink or apricot cream blush along the cheekbone itself, between the light and dark areas. Take the shape of your face into consideration (see overleaf).

blend

Using a medium-sized, soft buffing brush, blend everything together with small circular motions. The aim is to soften the edges, to connect and blend the different shades so they merge together for a flawless 3-D effect. If you need to intensify any areas, layer on a little more color and blend again. You can either do this with dark and light powders or you can add more cream foundation and then set it with a fine layer of translucent powder.

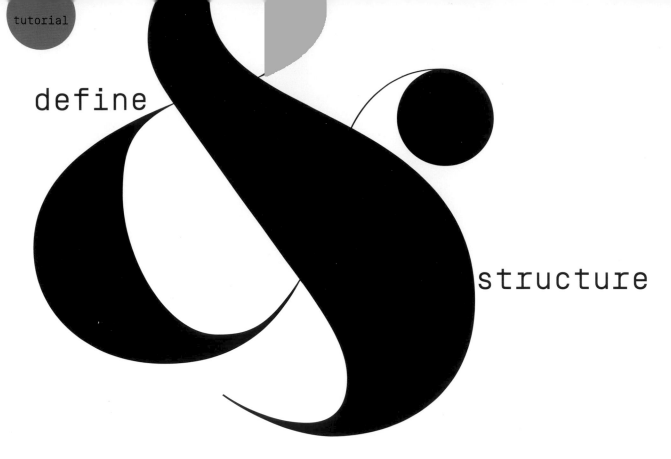

define & structure

Before contouring and highlighting or bringing any color and tone to the face, it's important to get to know your face shape and bone structure. Then you can decide what you need to do to make yourself look as fabulous as possible.

Thorough blending is essential for achieving a natural finish and although contouring takes practice, the results can be transformative.

The shape of a face dictates how make-up should be applied in order to enhance it in the best possible way. Contouring and highlighting techniques can then be used to define certain features and make others recede. Remember the principle: a darker shade is applied to make something recede, so it becomes less prominent, and a lighter shade is used to bring something forward, so the eye is drawn to it.

Once you have identified your face shape, you can use the following guidelines to help you apply make-up in the appropriate way to give your face more structure—for example, to bring out your cheekbones, to make your jowls recede and give your jawline more definition, or to make your nose look slimmer or shorter.

Identifying your face shape is easy to do. Simply take a long, hard look at yourself in a mirror. Assess the length and width of your face, the size of your forehead, the structure of your cheekbones, the size and shape of your chin and jaw. If you are struggling to see it, use an old lipstick or eye pencil to draw the outline of your reflection on the mirror. I have categorized the most common face shapes opposite to help you make the most of your features.

ROUND

This is a full face with soft, rounded curves, and the width and length are almost the same. Apply shading around the sides of the face to slim it down and under the cheekbones and jaw to cut them out, reduce fullness, and add structure. Highlight the center of the face to add length, and apply blush under the cheekbones but not on the apples themselves.

HEART

The face is widest at the forehead, strongly curving down to a pointed chin. Apply shading to make the forehead look smaller, the width of the face narrower, and the chin shorter and softer. Highlight under the eyes, the middle of the forehead, the bridge of the nose, and across the chin to add more width. Apply blush below the apples of the cheeks, starting at the hairline near the ear and blending it down.

SQUARE

The width is the same at the forehead, cheeks, and jawline, and roughly the same as the length from hairline to chin. The jawline is strong and angular and the forehead is broad. The aim is to minimize the width of the forehead and jaw, soften the hard angles, and bring out the cheekbones with shading, and to lengthen the face by highlighting under the eyes and down the center of the forehead, nose, and chin.

RECTANGULAR

The face is longer than wider, with quite straight sides and a broad, square jaw. The aim is to use shading to soften the hard lines and angles, creating a smaller, softer jaw, and to bring out the cheekbones. Keep the highlighter to the central part of the face and under the eyes. Apply blush to follow the line of the contouring.

OVAL

Broader on the cheekbones and narrower on the forehead and chin, this balanced face shape is seen as the ideal. Minimal contouring is needed, so just apply shading and highlighting where shadow and light naturally fall on your face to emphasize your great bone structure and bring it out even more, and use blush to accentuate your cheekbones and bring warmth to your face.

LONG

This face shape is long and slim, so the aim is to reduce length and add width and fullness. Apply shading around the hairline and chin to shorten the forehead and make the chin appear less pointed. Highlight the center of the forehead, the bridge of the nose, and under the eyes. Apply blush and highlighter to the apples of the cheeks to accentuate width and fullness.

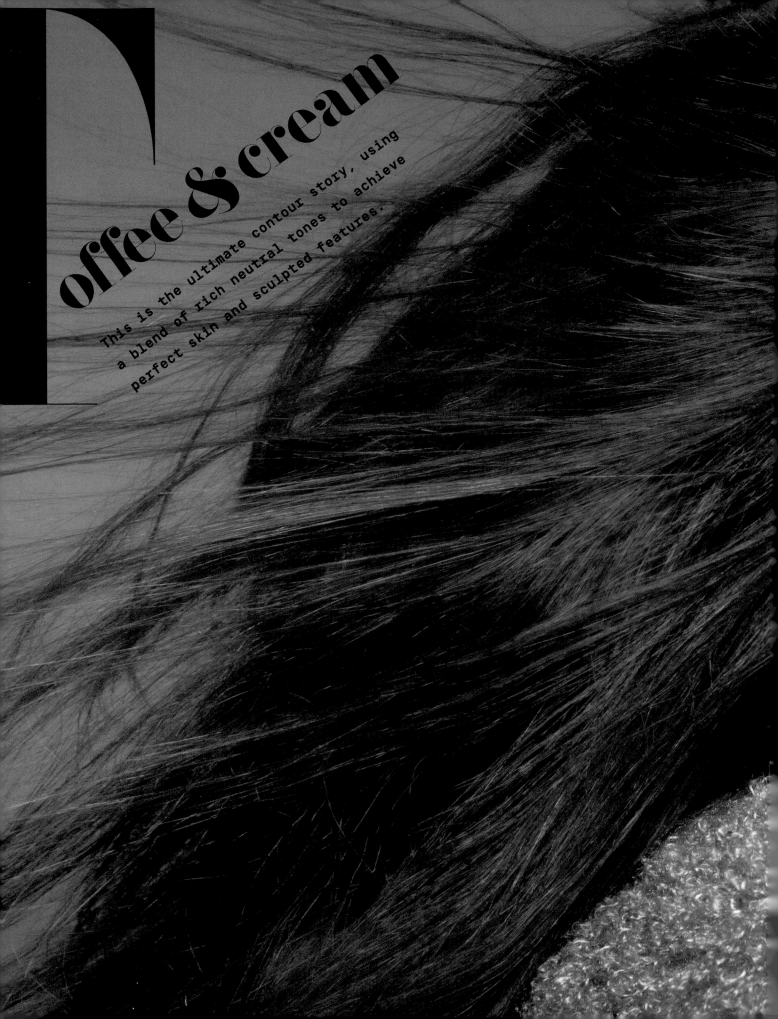

Coffee & cream

This is the ultimate contour story, using a blend of rich neutral tones to achieve perfect skin and sculpted features.

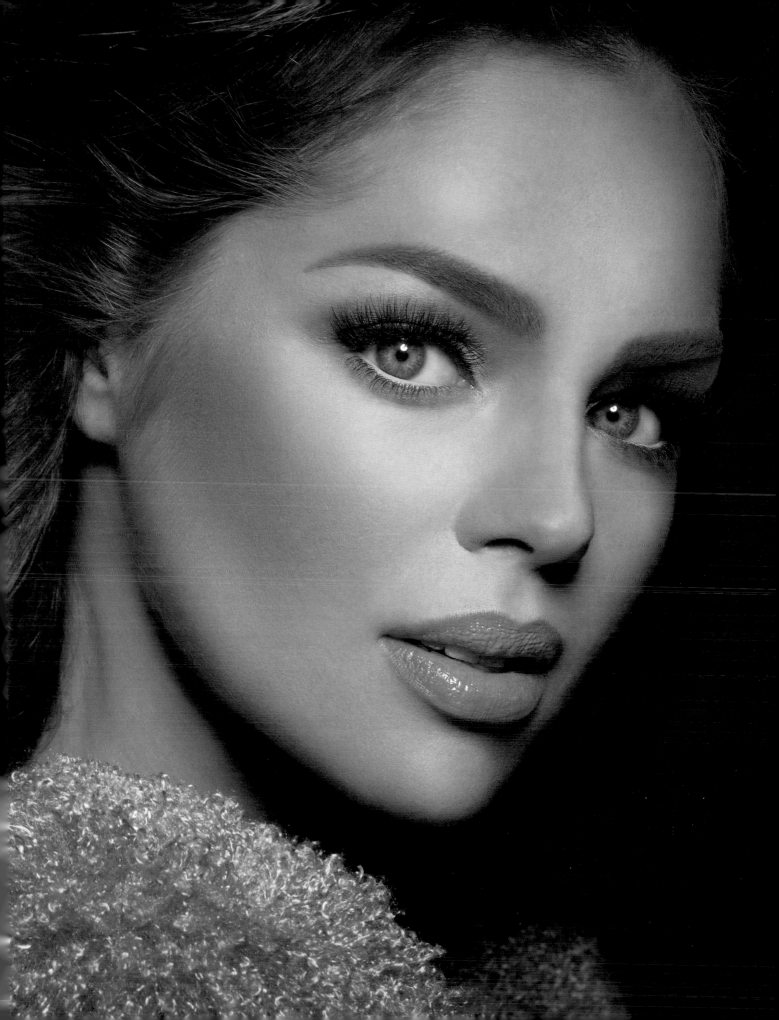

Toffee and Cream Transformation

This is a luxurious, expensive make-up look, where the aim is to have a glowing, luminous complexion with the features defined in a bespoke mix of toffee and cream shades chosen to flatter the skin—think sumptuous honey, mocha, chocolate, coffee, and vanilla. These are softly blended together to create areas of light and shade for a sculpted, polished, grown-up finish. Most people of any age can wear this make-up—the key is to choose shades that work well with your skin tone. It especially suits black, Latino, and yellow-toned skin, but is harder to do successfully on anyone with very cool undertones. Our model [previous spread] has pale olive skin, so I used a rich blend of warm caramels, creams, and peachy nudes. For the transformation on Andrea, I chose toffee shades with reddish undertones to bring out the warmth in her skin, with rich gold highlights to give it a glossy, soft-focus sheen. It's important to prime the face first, as the skin needs to be as smooth as possible for a perfect finish that will last. A layer of liquid foundation evens out the skin tone and provides a good base for blending the contouring creams, which are applied to give the face structure and definition.

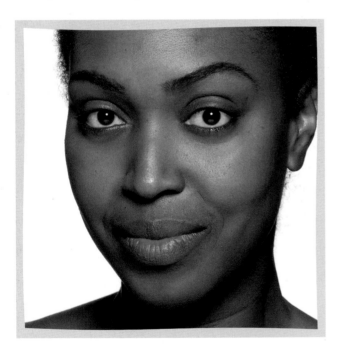
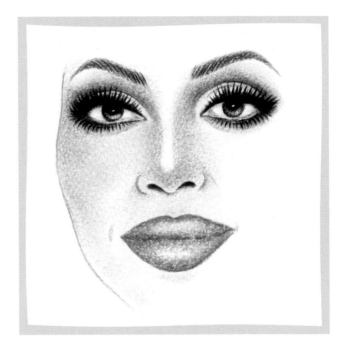

In her late forties, Andrea had never experienced contouring and was a bit scared of the idea, but I was determined to prove how powerful it can be. When I first started, she thought I was mad and was really sceptical that it would work, but she was over the moon with the end result.

face
Lightweight liquid foundation to match the skin tone.
Darker and lighter cream foundation for contouring.
Two shades of powder for contouring.
Dark apricot powder blush (1).
Gold-toned pigment (2).

eyes
Mid-brown matte brow powder.
Vanilla shimmery powder eyeshadow (3).
Rich, warm, toffee-colored powder eyeshadow (4).
Black gel eyeliner (5).
Dark brown matte powder eyeshadow (6).
Black mascara.
Lash clusters.
Vanilla pencil eyeliner (7).

lips
Soft brown lip pencil (8).
Lighter toning shade of nude-brown lip pencil (9).
Creamy caramel lipstick (10).
Lip gloss.

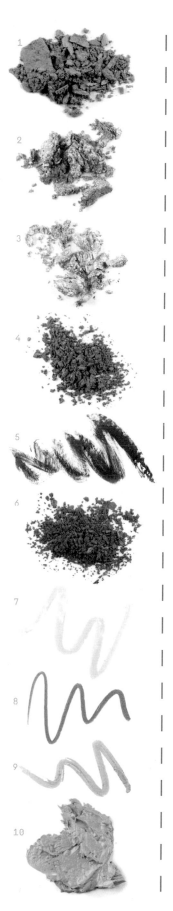

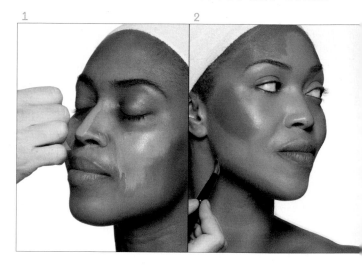

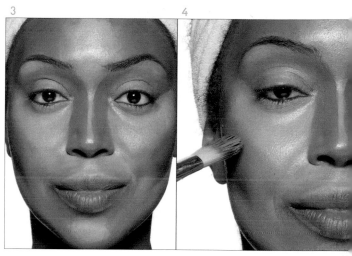

■face

1 When I'm color-matching foundation on black skin, I usually choose a shade one tone lighter, as it tends to look darker once it's on the skin. After prepping and priming (see pages 28–9), I applied a light, liquid foundation all over her face and blended it well to even out the skin tone.

2 Next, I contoured her face to give it more structure and definition (see pages 56–61). First, I applied the darker cream foundation on the areas where I wanted to create shadow— under the cheekbones to carve out their shape, under the jaw to define the jawline, at the sides of the temples to make the forehead look smaller, and down the sides of the nose to slim it down.

3 Then I added the lighter cream foundation to the areas that I wanted to draw attention to and brighten—under the eyes, in the center of the forehead, under the corners of the mouth and nose, in the center of the chin, on the bridge of the nose, and above the upper lip.

4 I blended the two colors into each other so they merged seamlessly, creating a 3-D effect.

5 To set the contouring creams and exaggerate the effect more, I polished the face with two shades of powder, applying the darker shade over the darker cream and the lighter powder over the lighter cream. I also applied a dark apricot powder blush to the apples of her cheeks to bring warmth to the face.

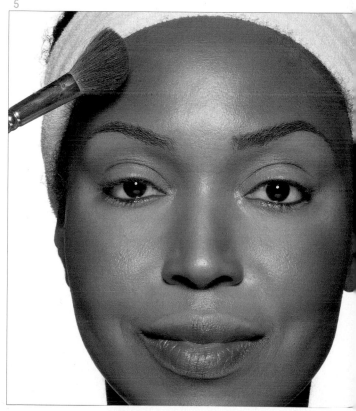

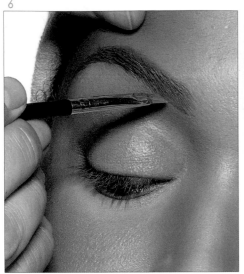

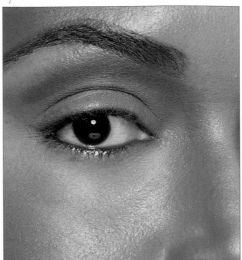

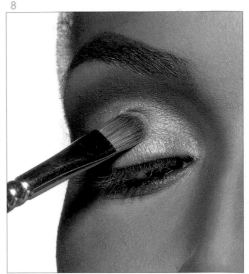

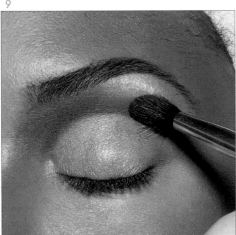

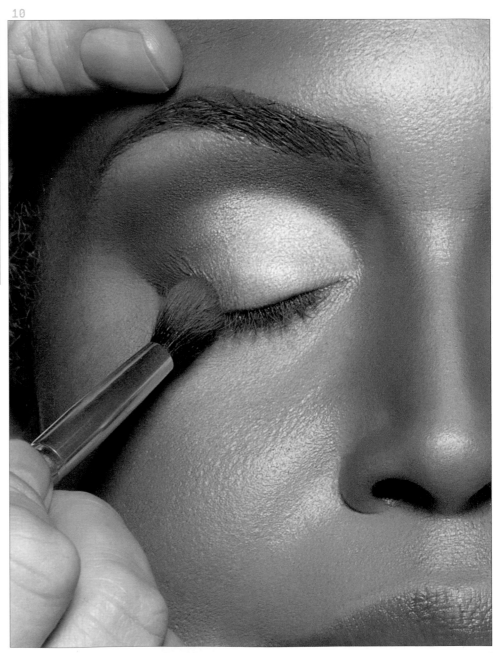

◼eyes

6 Andrea's eyebrows were already a good shape, so I just neatened them and filled in any gaps with mid-brown matte brow powder using a small angled brush and feathery strokes. It's important not to make the eyebrows too dark, as they can overpower and harden the face.

7 I used the dark contouring powder to carve out a socket crease, following the contour of the eye but drawing the line just above the natural socket. I extended this at the inner corner of the eye, sweeping it down the side of the nose to exaggerate the slimming effect of the facial contouring.

11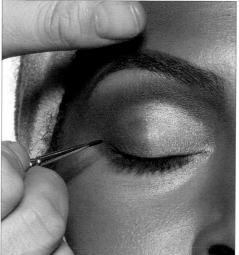

12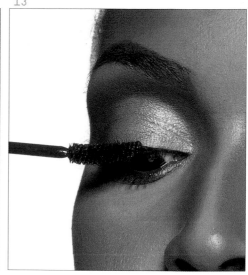

13

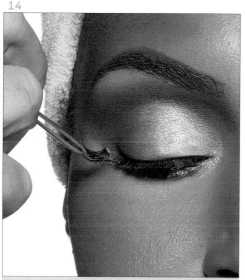

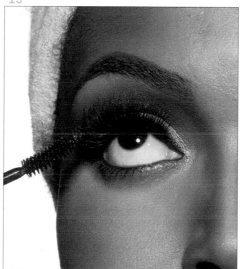

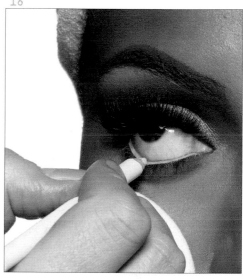

14

15

16

Pro trick

You can create your own lash clusters by cutting a full strip into four or five sections. Remember which are the outer and inner edges of the lashes and apply them in the correct order, working from the outer corner of the eye inward and leaving a little gap between each cluster. Breaking the lashes up gives a more natural effect but still creates the desired fullness.

8 I applied a shimmery vanilla powder eyeshadow to the main part of the eyelid, around the tear duct, and under the brow bone.

9 I then emphasized the socket crease even more using a rich, warm, toffee-colored powder eyeshadow.

10 I took this color onto the outer corner of the eyelid and blended it together with the vanilla shade.

11 I then swept it underneath the eye from the outer corner and blended everything together for a rich, warm, chocolaty look.

12 I lined the upper lash line with black gel liner and smudged a little dark brown matte eyeshadow over

the top for a softer finish; this creates a natural-looking shadow above the lash line.

13 I curled the upper lashes and applied black mascara from roots to tips, for thickness and fullness.

14 Then I added clusters of false lashes where they were needed to give a natural, fluttery look.

15 I added more mascara to the roots of the lashes only, to create more depth without making them look too heavy and unnatural.

16 I finished the eyes by applying vanilla pencil eyeliner inside the waterline to give her a fresh, wide-awake look.

> *"When Gary started the contouring, I really couldn't imagine what the end result would be, but it looked amazing. The combination of light and shadow really brought out the best in my face and gave my skin a luminous glow."*

■lips

17 First, I primed her lips with foundation to mask any natural pigment, as I didn't want it to show through the lipstick and alter the color.

18 I outlined her lips with a soft brown pencil to perfect the shape, taking the color a little way in to add depth.

19 I then applied a slightly lighter toning lip pencil over the lips, blending the color inward but keeping the central part of the lips bare. Applying two graduating tones of brown pencil as a basecoat gives the lips a 3-D effect.

20 I then applied a creamy, caramel lipstick with a lip brush over the entire mouth, so the center of the lips, with no basecoat, is slightly lighter than the outer edges, giving the lips a really full pout.

21 I finished the lips with a hint of gloss in the center of the bottom lip.

As a final touch, I added some warm, gold-toned pigment to the beginning of her eyes, under the arch of her brows, and on the apple of her cheeks. This gives the skin a luxurious, soft-focus finish.

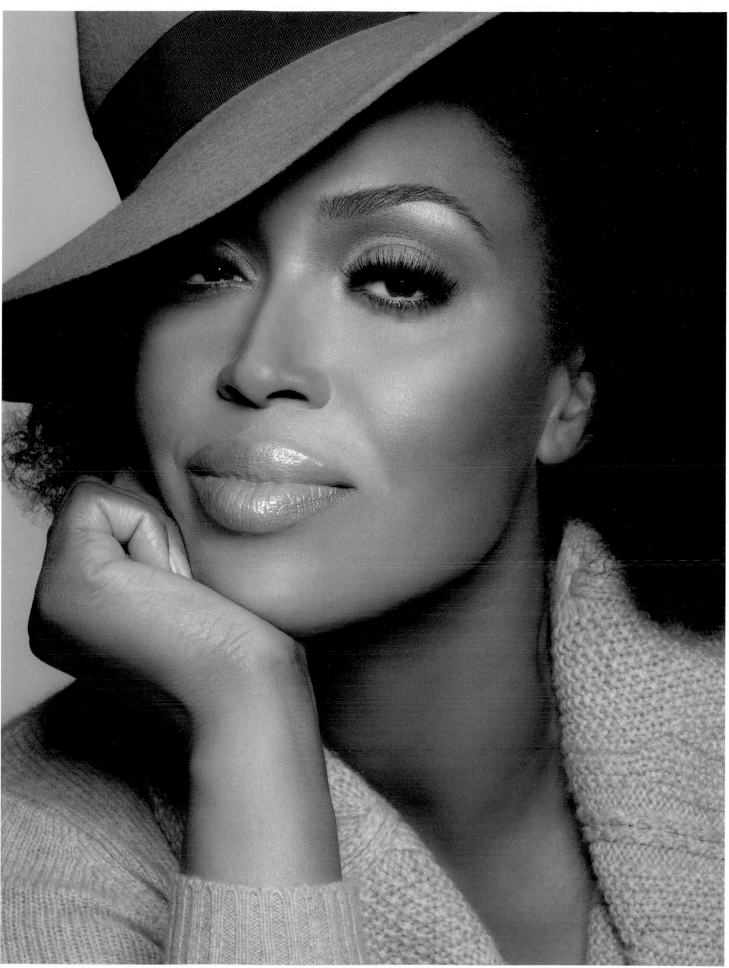

Powder

Powder is a make-up staple and it's definitely a product that I couldn't do without. I use it to set foundation, concealer, or contouring, to increase the make-up's staying power, to minimize or maximize shine [depending on whether it contains light-reflecting particles], and to protect the skin from fallout when I'm applying eye make-up. Powder can also help to even out skin tones.

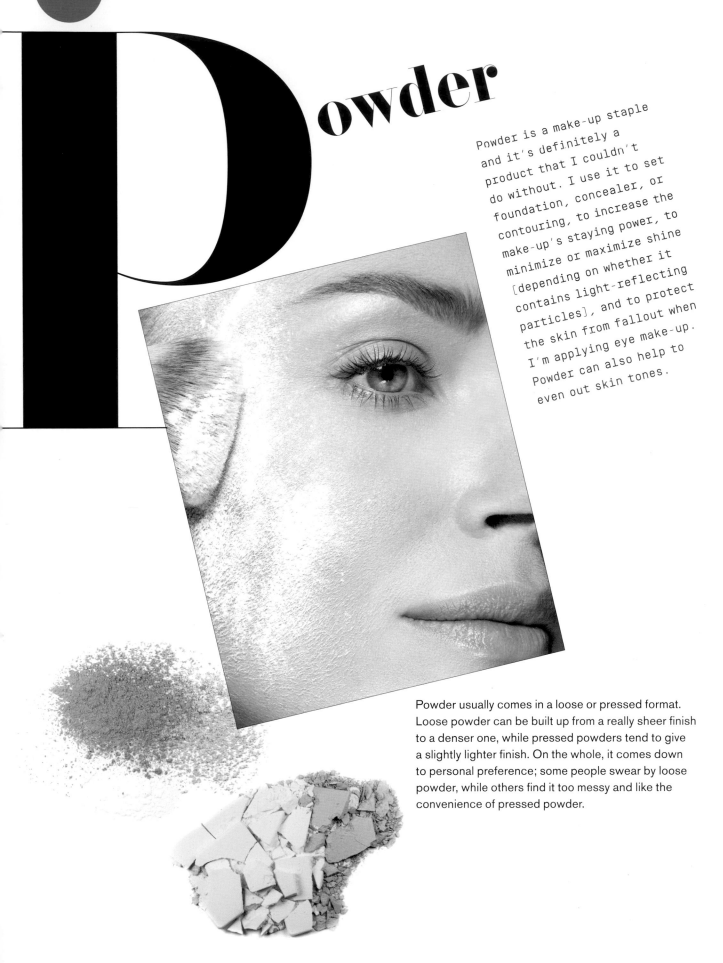

Powder usually comes in a loose or pressed format. Loose powder can be built up from a really sheer finish to a denser one, while pressed powders tend to give a slightly lighter finish. On the whole, it comes down to personal preference; some people swear by loose powder, while others find it too messy and like the convenience of pressed powder.

types of powder

The type of powder you choose depends on how you want to use it and the effect you want to achieve.

translucent powder This is a fine powder that imparts no color onto the skin. It is very versatile and is often dubbed the make-up artist's secret weapon. I mainly use this powder to set make-up, control shine, and make the blending of powder products (such as eyeshadow) easier.

foundation powder A foundation and powder in one, this offers more coverage and comes in many shades. It can be used for contouring and is often layered on top of liquid foundation to give it more staying power, but it can also be used on its own and is a great choice for those with oily skin. Use a tissue to blot the primer, moisturizer, or foundation first, as otherwise it can go patchy on application.

mineral powder This is formulated for sensitive skin and is easy to build up from sheer to heavier coverage.

light-reflective or sparkly powders These contain light-reflective or glittery particles that add radiance to the skin. The former are great for highlighting areas where light falls naturally; the latter are only for evening use.

how to apply

Use a fat, fluffy, natural-bristle brush of an appropriate size. You can use a larger brush for the bigger areas of the face—the forehead, planes of the cheeks, and the jawline, as well as the collarbones and décolletage—and a smaller one for the eyes and around the nose and mouth. Use sweeping, circular motions and concentrate on polishing the product into the skin, so it doesn't sit on the surface or settle into fine lines on the face, especially around the eye area and in the nose-to-mouth creases.

To apply loose powder, dip the tip of the brush into the powder. Then, holding the brush over the powder pot, tap off the excess before applying it to the face. If you want a very sheer, minimal coverage, sweep your brush over the T-zone only and blend it outward onto the cheeks. Always build up coverage gradually.

To apply pressed powder, sweep the brush around the compact a few times and apply it to the face. Alternatively, you can use the powder puff, simply pressing it gently onto the face where it's needed. You can control whether you create sheer or full-on coverage by how much pressure you apply when you push the puff into the skin.

Tips

» Apply powder in moderation, building it up gradually to the desired level of coverage—the skin won't look real if you cake it on.

» Always remove excess powder from your brush or puff before application to avoid build-up on the skin—tap, don't blow.

» For a more natural look, only powder areas that need it—such as on the T-zone to counteract shine.

» Dust a little powder over the eyelids before applying powder eyeshadow, as it will help the eyeshadow to blend more easily on the lids.

» If your eyeshadow is difficult to blend, add a little translucent powder.

» Don't overdo powder on dry or older skin, as it will lie in the lines and creases and age you even more. Be especially careful around the eyes. Powder will also accentuate dryness and flaky areas.

» If you've got oily skin, powder is your number-one must-have product. However, if the skin is really oily, the powder will clog and make your face look dirty, so use blotting paper or a tissue first to get rid of excess oil. I often blot the face after applying foundation and before I put any powder onto the skin.

» If you are going to use cream blush, apply it onto liquid or cream foundation before applying powder; if you are using powder foundation, use powder blush.

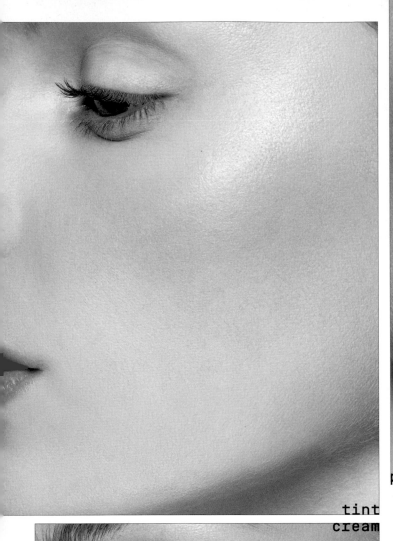

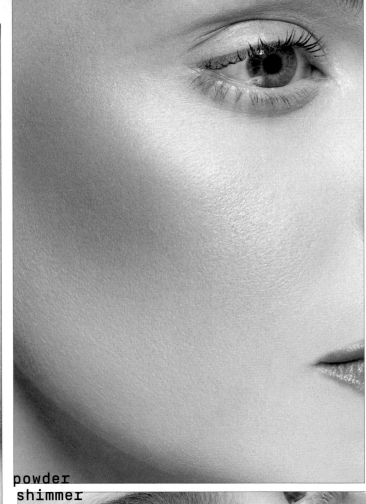

tint
cream

powder
shimmer

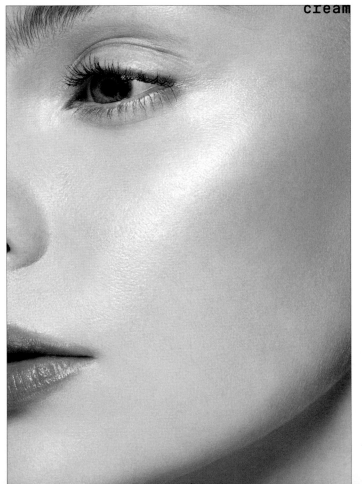

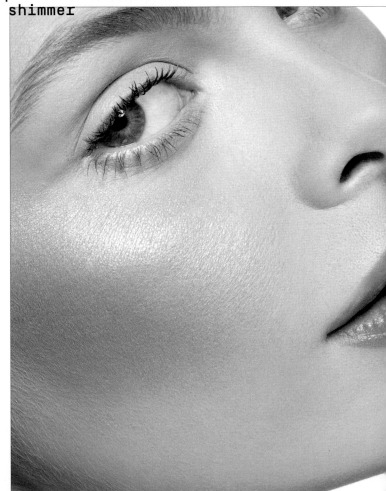

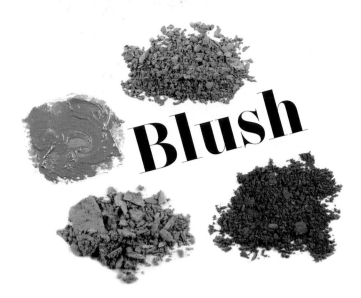

Blush

A flush of color on the cheeks exudes youth and vitality, and blush—whether powder, cream, gel, or liquid—adds warmth and brightness to the face. It enhances the cheekbones and really comes into its own when combined with contouring and highlighting.

With so many textures and shades to choose from—pinks, peaches, and apricots, bright fuchsias and corals, rich chocolates, caramels, maroons, and berry tones—it's important to pick the right blush for your skin and the occasion. Look for a color that complements your skin tone and texture, so the blush sits on the skin and looks believable. As a rule, the darker the skin, the more pigment it can take and the stronger the blush can be. Pinch your cheek gently and try to find a shade that matches the natural color of your skin. Bear in mind that your skin may be pale with cool undertones during winter and warmer in summer, and blush could then be combined with bronzer. The time of day is also a consideration, as you may be able to wear stronger colors in the evening than in the daytime, and you may prefer a powder finish with a matte or shimmery texture at night, but a dewy cream or sheer tint in the day.

For light skin, try soft pastels, petals, pinks, and corals. For medium skin, try warm apricots, corals, bronzes, and browns. For dark skin, try berry colors, plums, and fuchsias.

how to apply

Apply powder blush with a soft-bristle brush; it's easy to overload the brush, so I often use one to apply and another to blend. Don't use brushes that are too big. A medium-sized angled brush cut for the face is ideal for application, then use a feathery brush to blend. Sweep it softly up and down the mid-planes of the cheeks and use circular motions on the apples. If the color is too intense, dust translucent powder over it and blend. Always apply blush in moderation, as it's easier to build up than take off if you overdo it.

Cream or gel blush can be dotted on the cheek and then blended outward using fingertips, a sponge, or a brush.

If your face is round, apply blush on the planes of your cheekbones and not on the center of your cheeks; keep it on the sides and mid-section, following the contour of your cheekbones. If your face is slim, apply blush to the apples of the cheeks to fill them out. Use blush to warm up the temples, the bridge of the nose, the chin, and décolletage.

tint Usually in the form of a gel or fluid, tints or stains are possibly the trickiest blushes to apply because they dry quickly, so you have to place the product accurately and blend it with speed. The colors can be hard to gauge, as they often come out either too sheer or too intense, compared to what you see in the tube. On the plus side, they last all day, are water-resistant, and give a fresh, sheer glow.

powder Probably the most universal type of blush, powder is easy to apply and you can make it look very natural or build it up for greater intensity. A matte texture gives the densest, boldest color; shimmery or light-reflective blush diffuses when it hits the skin, giving a softer finish. Powder blush looks great on oily skin and is quite long-lasting, but it doesn't last as long as cream or tint blushes.

cream Always apply cream blush before powder and don't use it over powder foundation, as it will look blotchy and dirty. Cream blush gives concentrated color, so apply it sparingly and take extra care to blend it well using your fingertip, a sponge or a fiberoptic brush. Cream blush gives a dewy finish, which is nice for the daytime, and it is moisturizing for dry or older skin.

shimmer More suitable for the evening, shimmer blush, which contains light-reflective particles, offers a quick way to give a healthy, radiant glow to the cheeks, acting as a blush and highlighter in one. Apply it in the same way as powder blush to accentuate the high planes of the face that you want to brighten and bring forward—but use sparingly, as you don't want to make the face too sparkly.

Bronzer

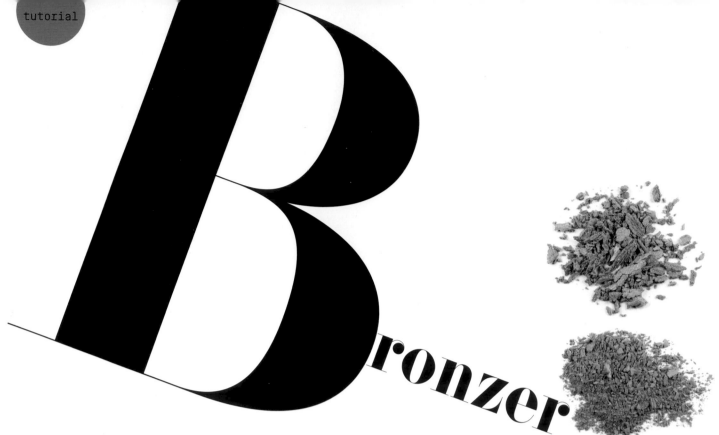

We all love a holiday and most of us enjoy relaxing in the sun, but while a light tan may make us feel glowing and healthy [sunlight stimulates the production of Vitamin D], we are now fully aware of the damage that it can cause to our skin. With all the great make-up products designed to give us a natural, sun-kissed look, why not fake it instead? Here, with her flawless skin and dazzling blue eyes, the gorgeous Chloe Green wears that golden glow to perfection.

To help give the skin that golden warmth of summer, choose a bronzer that's one or two shades darker than your natural skin tone in a light formula that won't conceal its radiance or create a mask-like finish. Look for a bronzer with a little golden shimmer or sheen for a soft, sun-kissed glow. I find powder bronzer gives a more natural effect than cream or liquid formulas; it's easier to control, as it blends well, letting you build up the intensity gradually—with liquid or cream bronzers, you can easily overdo it.

One of the most important things to remember is that bronzer is not for contouring. Most bronzers have an orange undertone and a light shimmer, or they contain light-reflecting particles. When you're contouring, you need a neutral tone and a matte finish to create shadow and enhance shape and form; a shimmery bronzer will have the opposite effect, reflecting light and highlighting.

Don't bronze your whole face; focus on where the light hits your face: your cheekbones, forehead, chin, nose, and ears, as well as down your neck and onto your shoulders, collarbones, and décolletage. If other parts of your body are going to be on view, don't forget to give them a light tan to match—there are so many great wash-off gels and body lotions, as well as fake tans and professional spray tans, for a longer-lasting, all-over glow.

Tips

» On dark skin tones, bronzer works well if you mix it with blush, as this prevents it from looking ashy.

» On fair skin, a sheer bronzer with peach tones gives a subtle effect without looking unnaturally orange.

» Try to put bronzer on in daylight, as it's so easy to overdo it.

» A shimmery bronzer will highlight areas much more than a matte one— keep that in mind as you get older.

» Apply powder bronzer with a large, round, soft blending brush.

» If your skin is very dry, try a cream, gel, or liquid bronzer, which you can mix with a little moisturizer for a fresh and youthful look.

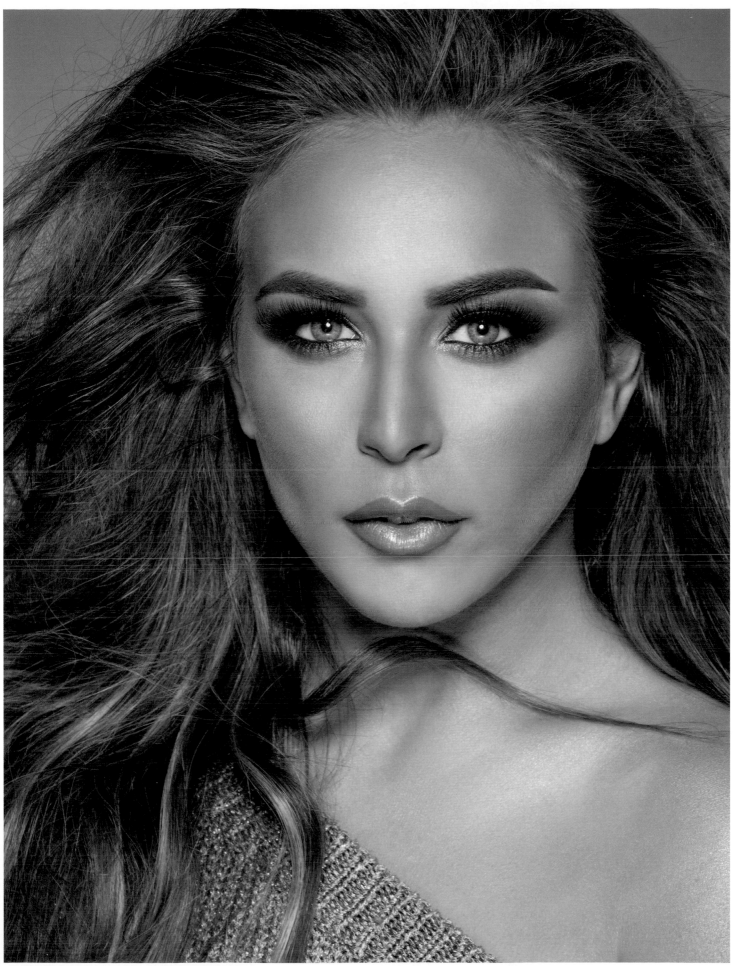

Sun-kissed Goddess

This look instantly transports me to the French Riviera and conjures up that wonderful glow on your skin after a day at the beach.

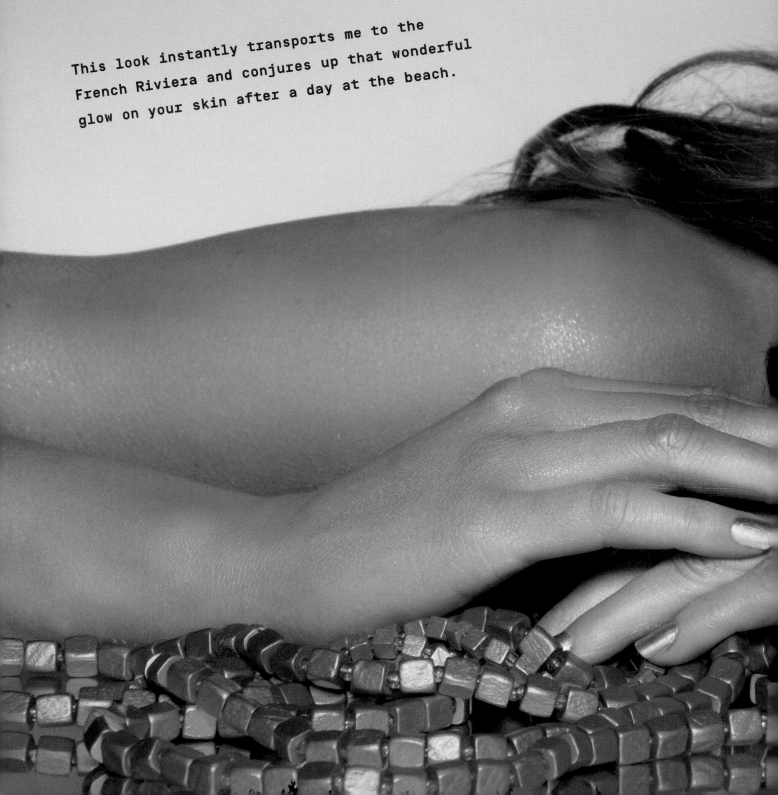

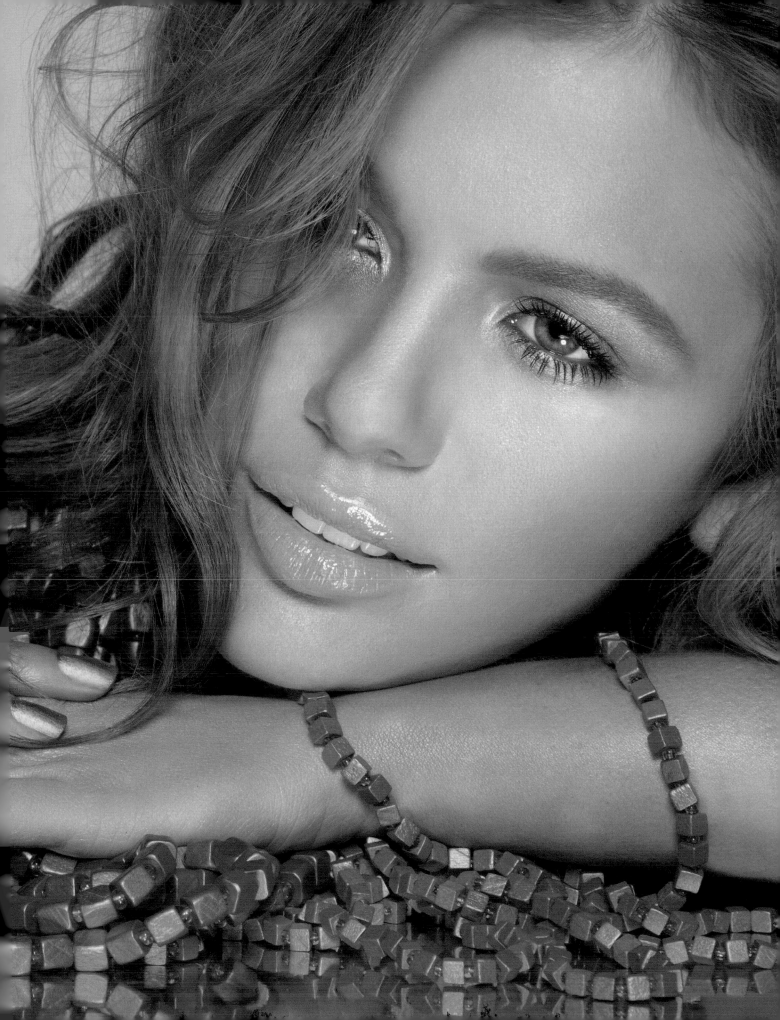

Sun-kissed Goddess Transformation

This is the ultimate glow story and you can almost feel the warmth of the sun on your face. The aim is to re-create that magical, golden light of long summer evenings as the sun is beginning to dip toward the horizon. Try to incorporate as many warm tones as possible onto your face, eyes, and lips, as they really lift the skin and make you seem to glow from within, while shimmering textures add a luxurious sheen and create a soft-focus effect that is flattering for all complexions. This make-up gives the healthy look that we all want in the summer and it looks glossy and fabulous on everyone—just remember to apply some fake tan to your body to tie the look together. On our model [previous page], I've shown a youthful, daytime look, where she seems to be bathed in golden sunlight, with lightly bronzed skin and shimmery gold textures on her eyes and lips. The transformation on Lynne shows an evening version, with rich bronze and antique-gold tones that bring out the hazel-green of her eyes and flatter her skin's warm undertones. I contoured her face to give it a little more structure and used slightly deeper colors to define her features, toning down the shimmer by blending it with matte eyeshadow and adding lip liner and a few false eyelashes.

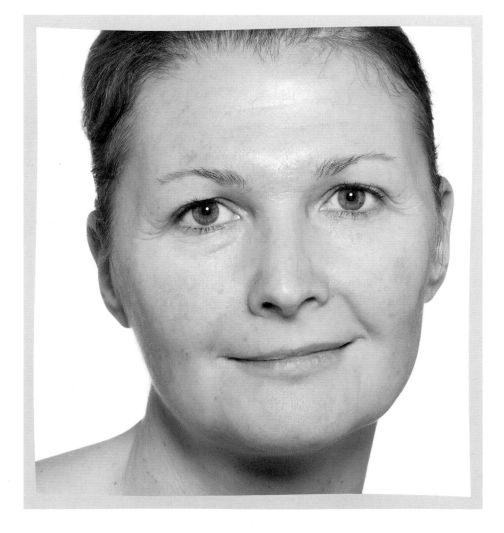

This is my beautiful sister Lynne. At 50, she was convinced she could no longer wear shimmer eyeshadow. I wanted to prove that if it's applied in the right place and in the right way, it's easy to wear and can look stunning on anyone.

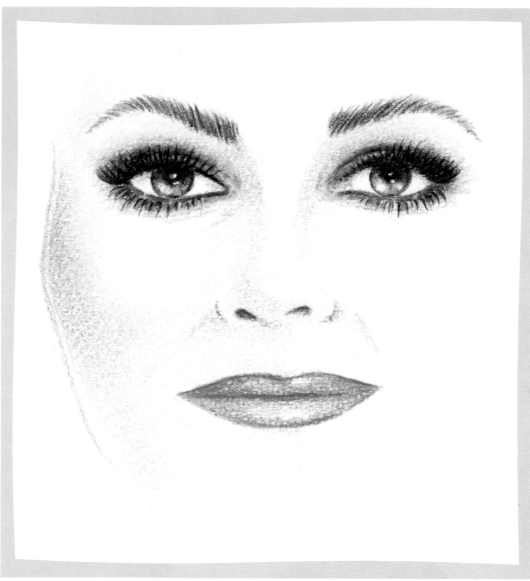

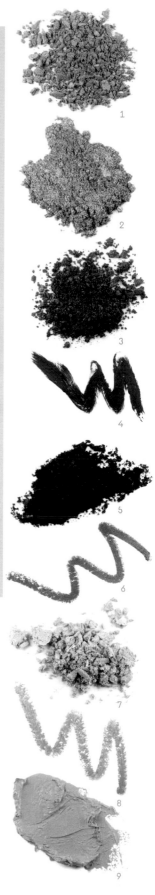

face

Hydrating, radiance-
boosting primer.
Liquid foundation to match
the skin tone.
Two shades of cream
foundation for contouring.
Contouring powders in the
same shades.
Warm apricot blush (1).

eyes

Matte brow powder
in a warm taupe.
Gold shimmer powder
eyeshadow (2).
Rich, rusty brown, matte
powder eyeshadow (3).
Black mascara.
Individual lashes and clusters
of false lashes.
Black gel eyeliner (4).
Black matte powder
eyeshadow (5).
Bronze eyeliner pencil (6).
Gold pigment (7).

lips

Creamy burnt-orange
pencil lip liner (8).
Creamy burnt-orange
lipstick (9).
Clear lip gloss.

1

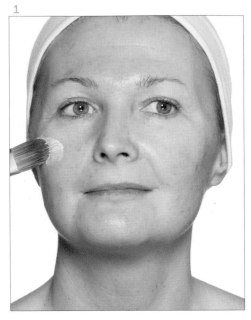

2

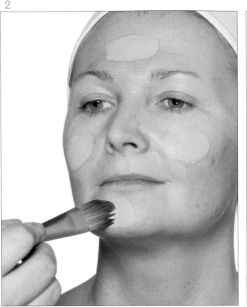

3

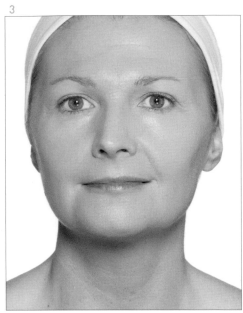

4

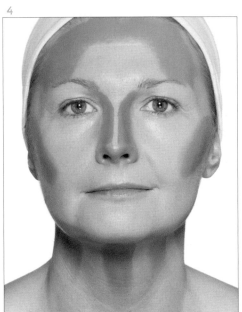

5

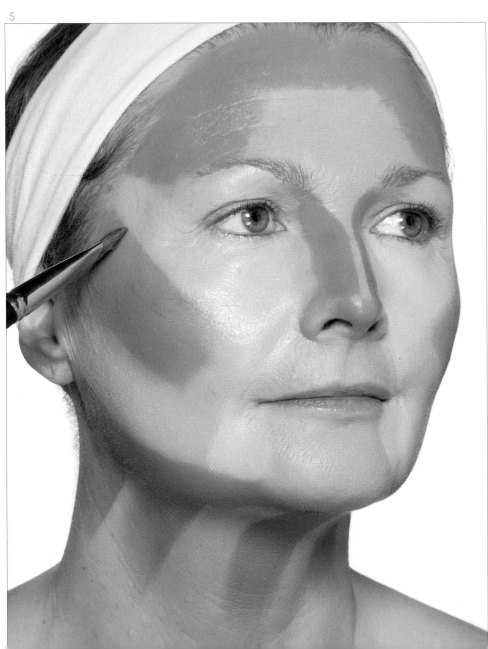

Blend the contouring gently, working a soft brush in small, circular motions to soften the edges without rubbing off the creams.

■face

1 After prepping the face, I applied a hydrating, radiance-boosting primer to create a good base.

2-3 Lynne had a slight tan, so I chose a yellow-toned liquid foundation. I applied it with a brush and blended it well to even out her skin tone.

4 If you are doing this look for the daytime or on young skin, you can sculpt the face with a matte powder bronzer and a shimmer powder highlighter, but I used two shades of cream foundation to help lift her face and create the illusion of more youthful skin (see page 56). I first applied the darker shade below the cheekbones to accentuate them, down the sides of the nose to slim it down, around the temples and the top of the forehead to make this area look smaller, and under the jaw to lift and define the jawline.

5 I applied the lighter shade under the eyes and below the corners of her mouth to lift and brighten those areas. Then I brushed a pinky apricot cream blush along the center of her cheeks, between the light and dark areas, to warm the skin and give it a summery freshness.

6 Using a clean buffing brush, I blended all these colors together to create a creamy, flawless finish.

7-8 To accentuate the sun-kissed glow and ensure a long-lasting finish—essential in a warm climate—I went over the cream foundations with contouring powders in the same shades, emphasizing the cheekbones and slimming the nose and jaw as before, and adding warmth to the face with apricot blush.

Tips

» A coral-orange lipstick will look fabulous with this look; it's a color that works well on anyone with lightly sun-kissed skin.

» Try an aqua-blue eyeliner on the waterline if you want to add more color to the look. It will intensify the color of blue and green eyes, and make brown and hazel eyes stand out more.

» Be careful where you place shimmer products around the eye area on older skin, as they will draw attention to any imperfections such as wrinkles and droopy lids, making them look heavy.

» Try to incorporate as many warm tones as possible, as they really lift the skin.

» Don't forget to bring any exposed areas of your body into the look—add a little shimmery powder to the skin to highlight the collarbones, décolletage, and shoulders.

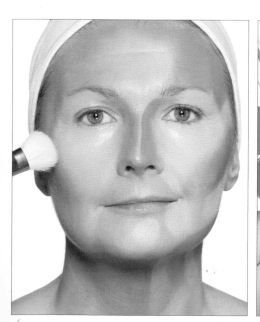

6

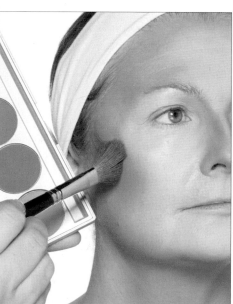

7

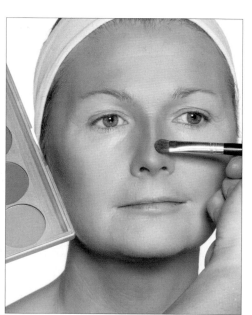

8

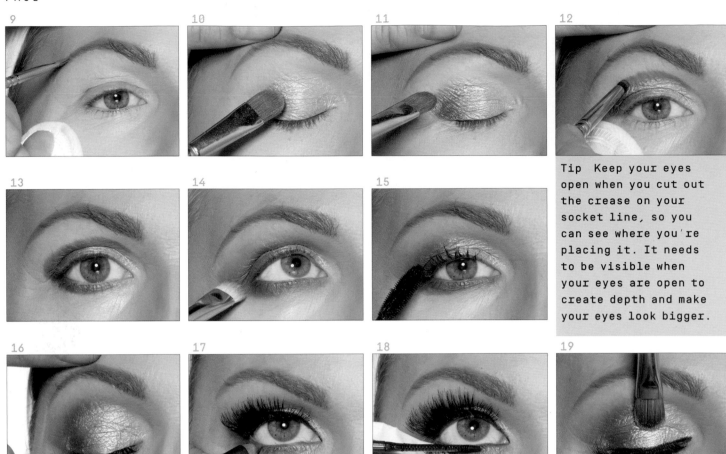

Tip Keep your eyes open when you cut out the crease on your socket line, so you can see where you're placing it. It needs to be visible when your eyes are open to create depth and make your eyes look bigger.

■ eyes

9 Lynne's eyebrows had been very overplucked so I went to town to make them look fuller. I chose a matte brow powder in a warm taupe, a shade lighter than her natural brows, to complement her skin tone and hair color. Using a small angled brush, I gradually built up the shape with light, feathery strokes to frame her face and make it look more youthful. Getting the tone and texture to look natural is the key—if you go too dark, it will harden the face.

10 Using a medium-sized brush, I applied gold shimmer eyeshadow to the main part of the eyelid, taking it into the natural socket crease and just underneath the eye at the inner corner.

11 I added a rich rusty brown matte eyeshadow to the outer corner and blended it into the shimmer powder on the lid to create more depth.

12 To combat the slight droop of her eyelids, I used a pencil brush and the same eyeshadow to cut out a crease just above the natural socket line, following its curve.

13 I swept the same color under the eye with an angled brush, taking it from the outer corner and fading it into the gold color at the inner corner.

14 Then I used a blending brush to soften all the edges and make the colors connect, with no hard lines.

15 I applied black mascara to the top lashes and let it dry before adding individual lashes and clusters of false lashes to add fullness, followed by another coat of mascara on the roots only to add depth. (The false lashes are optional and if you're doing this look for the daytime, don't go there.)

16 I lined the upper lash line with a black gel liner, keeping as close to the roots of the lashes as possible. Then

I smudged a little black eyeshadow over it, creating the impression of a shadow above the lash line, which makes the lashes look thicker.

17 To intensify the eye even more, I chose a burgundy-bronze eyeliner pencil and applied it to the waterline to make the green of her eyes pop. (Again, this is optional, and best saved for a more dramatic, nighttime look.)

18 I applied mascara to the lower lashes, holding a tissue under them to protect the skin from smudges.

19 To finish off the eye, I added a little gold pigment to the inner corner and to the very middle part of the lid, so the shimmer is visible when the eye is open. This catches the light, drawing attention to the eyes, and is great for an evening look. Using a smaller brush, I also added a touch of the shimmery pigment under the lower lash line at the inner corner of the eye.

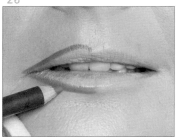

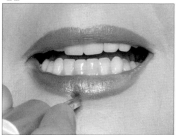

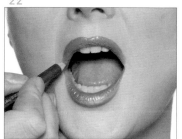

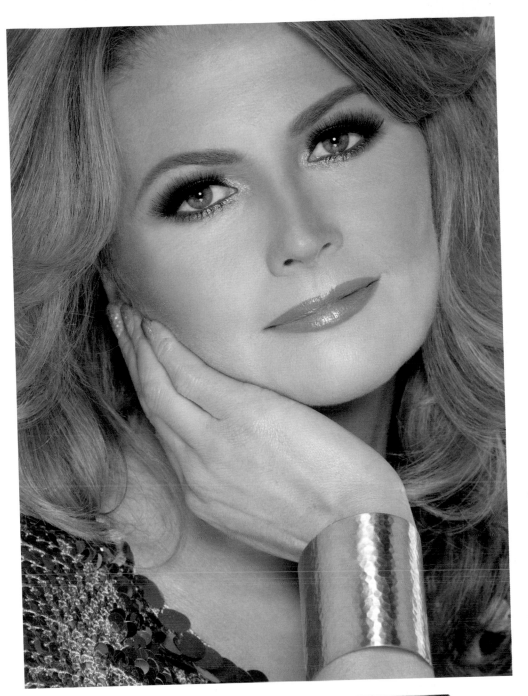

■ lips

20 As older lips tend to lose their plumpness, lining them just outside the natural outline makes them look fuller and prevents the lipstick from "bleeding" into fine lines around the mouth. I chose a creamy burnt-orange pencil to line her lips. Once I was happy with the shape, I colored in the lips to create a good base and give the lipstick more staying power.

21 I applied a creamy burnt-orange lipstick on top of the pencil, and then blotted it with a tissue and reapplied it. I repeated this a few times to give a longer-lasting finish.

22 I blended a little more of the pencil on top of the lipstick for a rich, 3-D effect. Finally, I added a dab of gloss in the middle of the bottom lip to catch the light.

"I was Gary's first muse when we were growing up and he's always known how to make me look beautiful, but I never imagined I could look like this at 50. I stopped wearing shimmer eyeshadow years ago because I thought I couldn't carry it off, but Gary showed me that by putting it in the right place I could. I don't lie in the sun much so it was great to learn how to create that glowing, sun-kissed look with make-up."

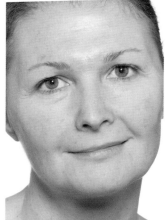

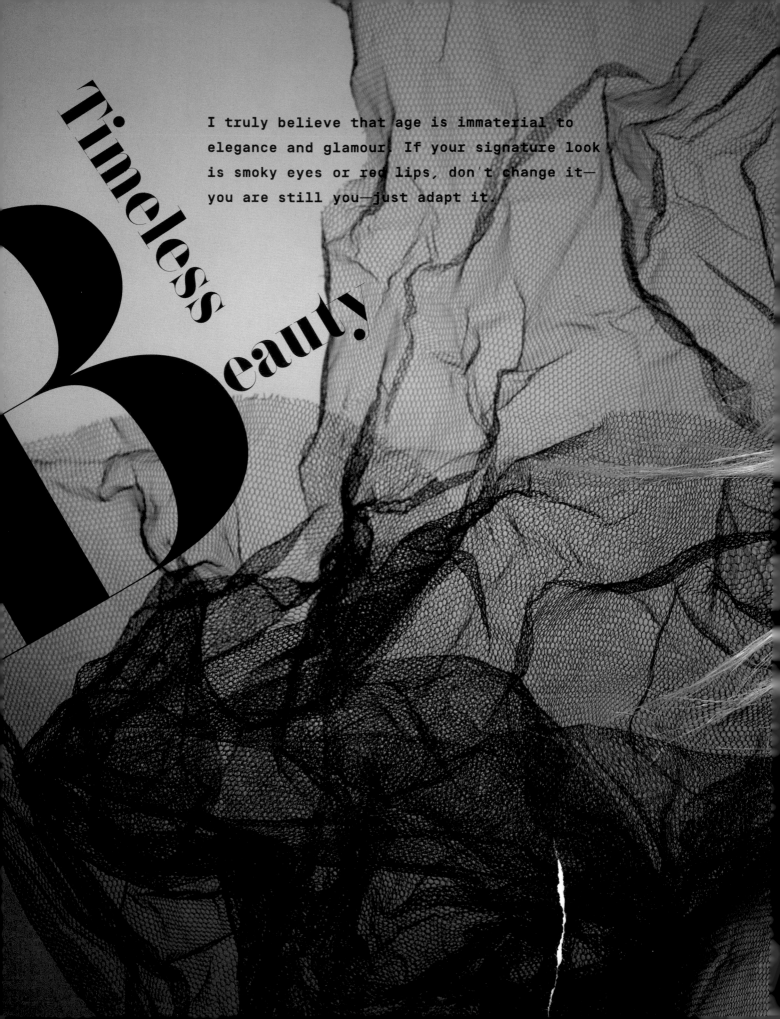

Timeless Beauty

I truly believe that age is immaterial to elegance and glamour. If your signature look is smoky eyes or red lips, don't change it—you are still you—just adapt it.

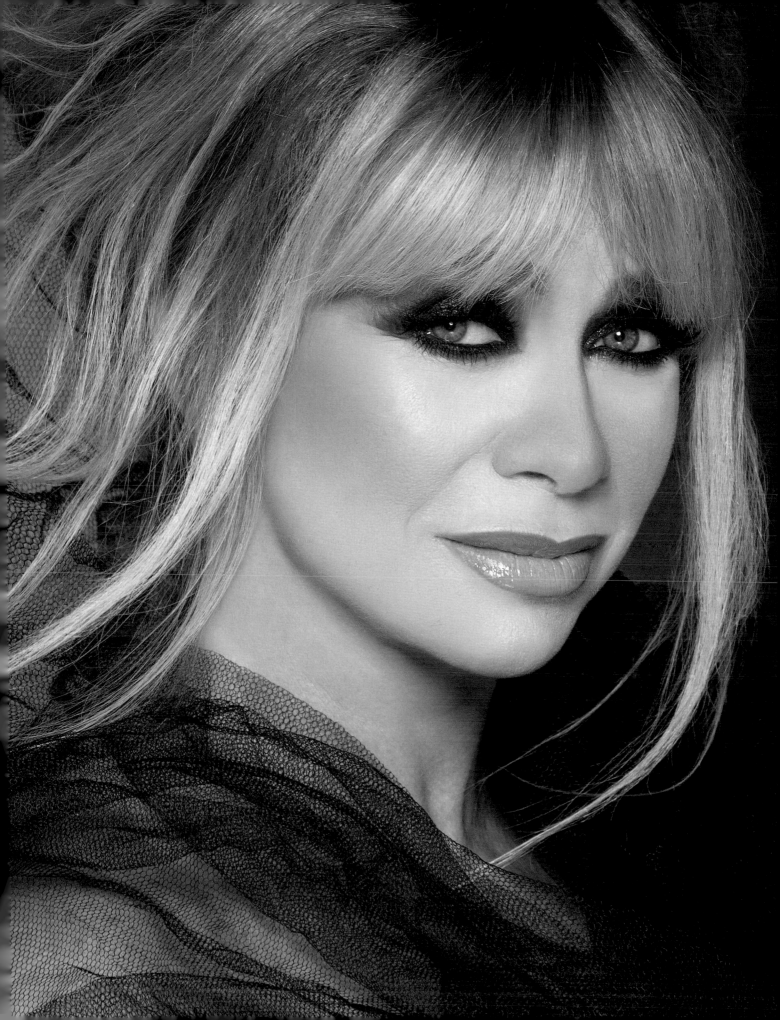

Timeless Beauty Transformation

Contrary to what many make-up pros teach, I don't necessarily believe that "less is more" when it comes to make-up on more mature ladies: it's a personal thing. As we age, the natural pigment in our face and hair fades, so I believe we should compensate for what we've lost and aim to put color and warmth back into the skin. When the contours of your face and the texture and tone of your skin have changed, the make-up you did 40 or even 20 years ago may no longer work for you, but so many women are stuck in a make-up rut, using the same shades, textures, and techniques as they did in their twenties. There is a wealth of clever products to be found

that can be used to add plumpness to lips and cheeks and restore glow and warmth to the skin. I have so much fun doing make-up for older clients and I really go to town to show them what is possible. The beautiful Jo Wood [previous page], who looks incredible at 60, is proof that glamour has nothing to do with age. A classic smoky eye with creamy nude lips looks stunning on her and suits her rock-chick persona. For Ann's transformation, I wanted to show her how amazing she could look in red lipstick. My motto is: try it and see, and if it looks good, do it. Never give up having fun with make-up and experimenting with new products.

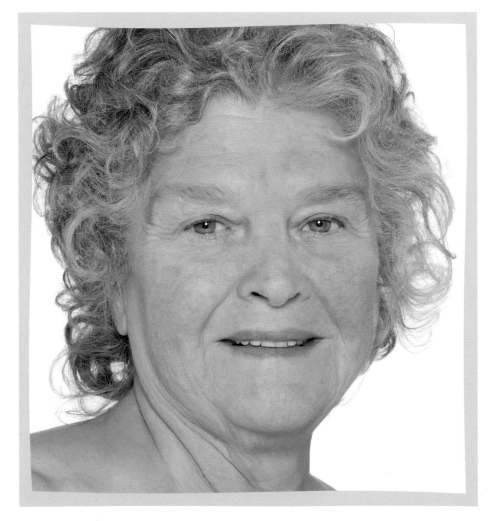

My mother, Ann, doesn't wear much make-up and, at 74, she wouldn't think of wearing red lipstick, but it's a great way to bring drama to the face and I wanted to prove that women of any age can wear it—as long as they take precautions against the color "bleeding" into lines around the mouth.

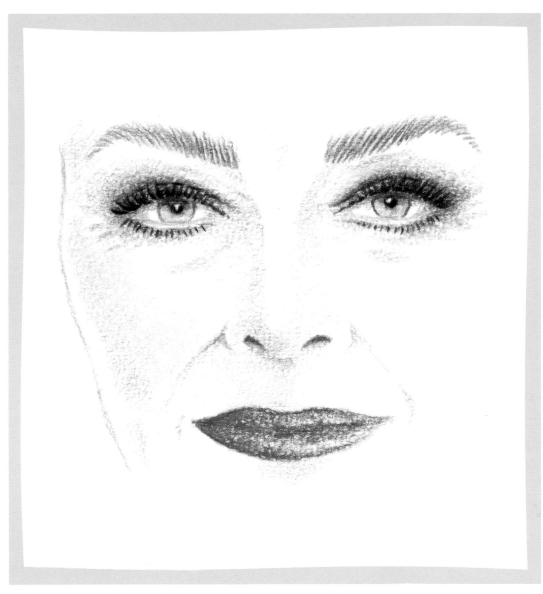

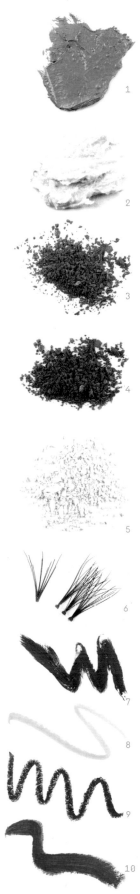

face

Yellow and green color
correctors.
Lightweight liquid foundation
to match the skin tone.
Two shades of cream
foundation for contouring.
Translucent powder.
Apricot cream blush (1).
Cream highlighter (2).

eyes

Ashy taupe matte
brow powder.
Soft brown eyeshadow
with a warm undertone
and a slight shimmer (3).
Slightly darker brown
eyeshadow in a similar tone
but with a matte finish (4).
Light bone-colored matte
eyeshadow (5).
Black mascara.
Individual lashes and lash
clusters (6).
Black gel eyeliner (7).
Creamy nude eyeliner
pencil (8).

lips

Creamy red lip pencil in the
same tone as the lipstick but
a shade deeper (9).
Cherry-red satin lipstick (10).

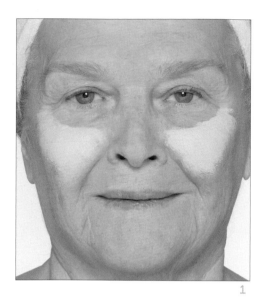

1

■face

1 After prepping Ann's face (see pages 28–9), the first thing I did was address the skin tone. Her skin is really good for her age but she does suffer from rosacea (enlarged facial blood vessels, which give a flushed appearance) and a few broken capillaries on the planes of her cheeks, so I used yellow and green color correctors to cancel out the redness (see pages 30–1).

2 First, I applied a lightweight liquid foundation all over her face to create a good, even base for blending the contouring creams. Then I started to contour her face using two shades of cream foundation, one two shades lighter than her natural skin tone and one two shades darker (see pages 56–61).

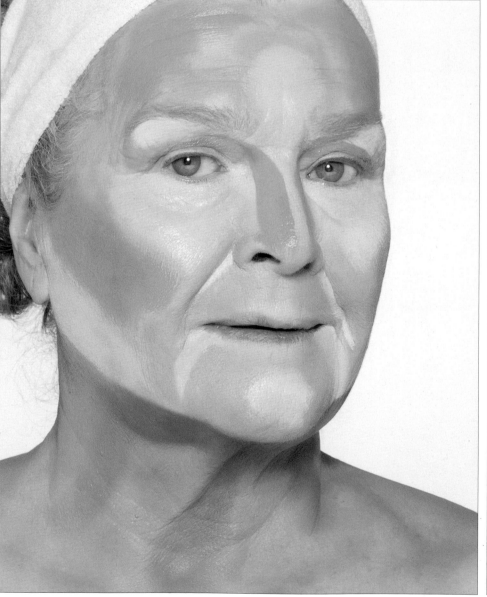

2

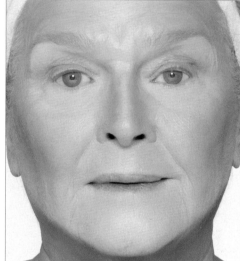

3

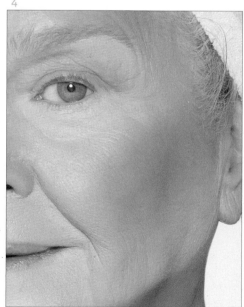

4

As usual, I applied the darker color where I wanted to create shadow and depth—under the jaw and chin, down the neck, in the hollows of the cheeks to cut out the cheekbones, down the sides of the nose to slim it, under the tip of the nose to lift it, in the crease of the eyes to define them, and around the temples and hairline to make this area recede. I then applied the lighter color to the areas I wanted to bring forward— under the eyes, above the cheekbones, below the brow bone, on the center of the eyelids and forehead, down the center of the nose, along the nose-to-mouth creases, under the corners of the mouth, in the middle of the chin, and on the collarbones. I used a large angled brush for the larger areas and a smaller brush for around the nose, eyes, and mouth, using a different one for each color of foundation.

3 I used a soft blending brush to combine the contours together to create a creamy, 3-D complexion with a lifted face and jawline. I then set the make-up with translucent powder, concentrating on the T-zone as I didn't want to make the face too matte—a light shine keeps the skin looking more natural than mask-like.

4 I added warmth to the face by applying an apricot cream blush to the apples of her cheeks. Then I applied a small amount of cream highlighter along the top of her cheekbones and on the beginning of the eye area to bring her face alive.

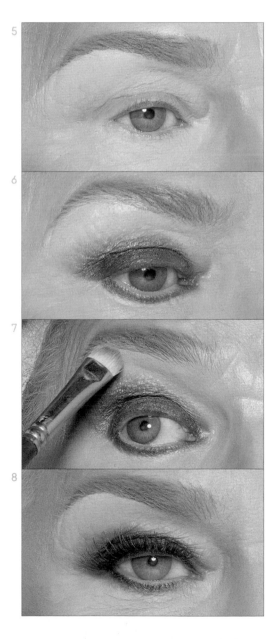

■ eyes

5 Eyebrows tend to get thinner and lose their color with age and eyelids start to sag, so the aim is to lift the eye area and create as much space as possible around the eyes. Having plucked and neatened any stray hairs, I used an ashy taupe brow powder and a small angled brush to fill in any sparse areas and create a nice arch.

6 I wanted to avoid anything that would make her face look sallow, so I chose a soft brown eyeshadow with red undertones and a slight shimmer, which really made the most of her lovely blue eyes. I concentrated the eyeshadow on the main part of the lid, taking it just up to the crease, and then added a slightly darker brown in similar tone but with a matte finish on the outer corners of the eyes and in the crease, and blended the two together. From the outer corners, I swept the shadow underneath the eyes with a round pencil brush, taking it just past halfway and blending it to nothing toward the inner corners.

7 I added a light bone-colored matte eyeshadow just underneath the brow bone to subtly highlight that area and lift the arch of the brow, opening up the eyes.

8 I curled the upper lashes and applied a small amount of black mascara before filling in any sparse areas with individual lashes and lash clusters, working from the outer edge to the middle of each eye. I then applied a fine black gel liner along the base of the upper lash line and smudged it so it wasn't too hard. This creates depth and makes the lashes look fuller. To brighten and open up her eyes, I applied a creamy, nude eyeliner pencil along the lower waterlines. Then I finished the eyes by applying a small amount of mascara to the bottom lashes.

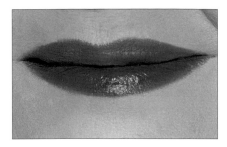

■lips

9 I started by priming her lips—you can just use the bit of foundation that's left on your brush. This makes lipstick last longer and neutralizes any natural pigment so the color is truer to the tube when it hits the mouth. I chose a cherry-red satin lipstick that works well against a warm skin tone and lined the lips with a soft lip pencil in the same tone but a shade deeper. I blotted the lips with a tissue and applied another coat of lip liner, this time taking the color into the center of the lips too, and blotted again. As well as helping to prevent the lipstick from "bleeding," this creates a stain and makes the color last longer. I then applied the lipstick over this with a brush, and blotted, reapplied, and blotted again. The darker shade of the pencil on the outer part of the lips creates a 3-D effect that makes the lips look fuller. Instead of using gloss, which is best avoided on older lips because it travels, I applied one last coat of the satin lipstick and didn't blot it to leave a light sheen on the lips. (See also pages 188–93 and 200 for more on red lipstick.)

Tips

face
» Contouring acts like a mini facelift, lifting the brows, chin, and jaw, and pulling out the cheekbones to add structure.

» Cream foundation is good for contouring older skin, as it gives a soft, milky complexion, whereas powder tends to settle into wrinkles.

» When applying powder on older skin, try to "push" it into the skin using a soft, rounded brush, so it doesn't settle in the lines.

» Setting contouring creams with translucent powder gives a soft effect, which I recommend for older skin, but for a more defined look, you can use two shades of powder to enhance and exaggerate the highlighted and shaded areas, matching the colors as above.

eyes
» Shimmery textures draw attention to lines so you need to be careful where you apply them on older skin, but a little shimmer lifts the face and keeps everything from looking too matte and chalky.

» Full strip lashes look too heavy on older faces, whereas individual lashes or lash clusters can be used to fill in any gaps and give a natural, youthful look.

» Applied to the lower waterline, nude pencil eyeliner in a shade that matches the skin brightens tired or red eyes—avoid anything too white, as it looks harsh and unnatural.

lips
» Lipstick with a satin finish is a good choice for older women, as gloss is high-maintenance and tends to "bleed," and matte can look hard.

» Lips tend to lose their fullness with age, so contouring the lips—by applying a darker shade on the outer edge, blending to a slightly lighter shade in the middle [see pages 190-3]— is a good trick, as it draws the eye and makes the lips look fuller and plumper.

» Blotting with single-ply tissue between multiple applications of lipstick helps to set the color as a stain and creates depth.

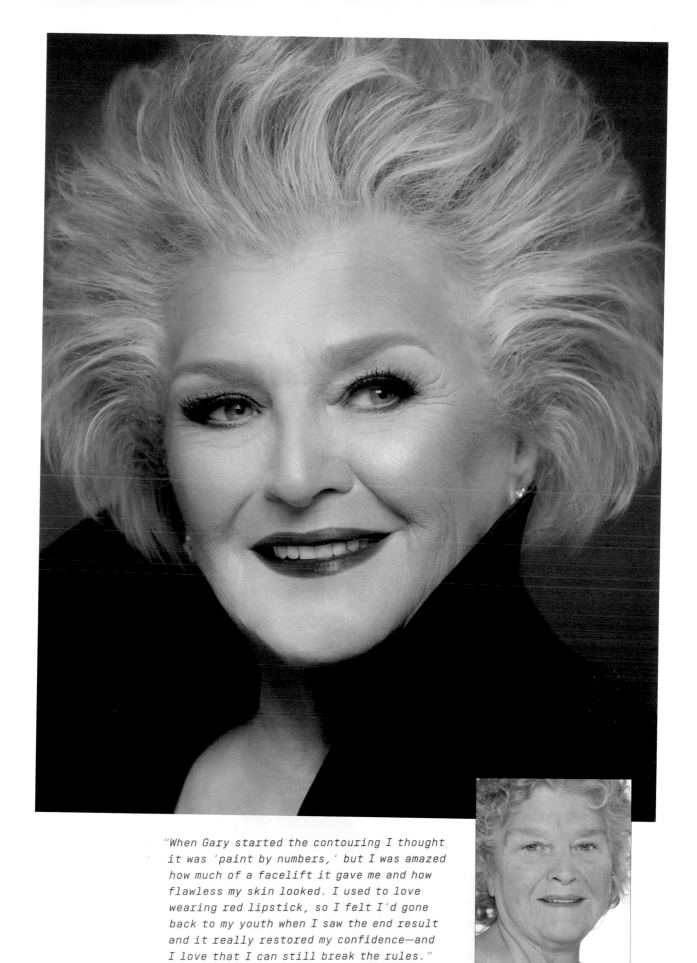

"When Gary started the contouring I thought it was 'paint by numbers,' but I was amazed how much of a facelift it gave me and how flawless my skin looked. I used to love wearing red lipstick, so I felt I'd gone back to my youth when I saw the end result and it really restored my confidence—and I love that I can still break the rules."

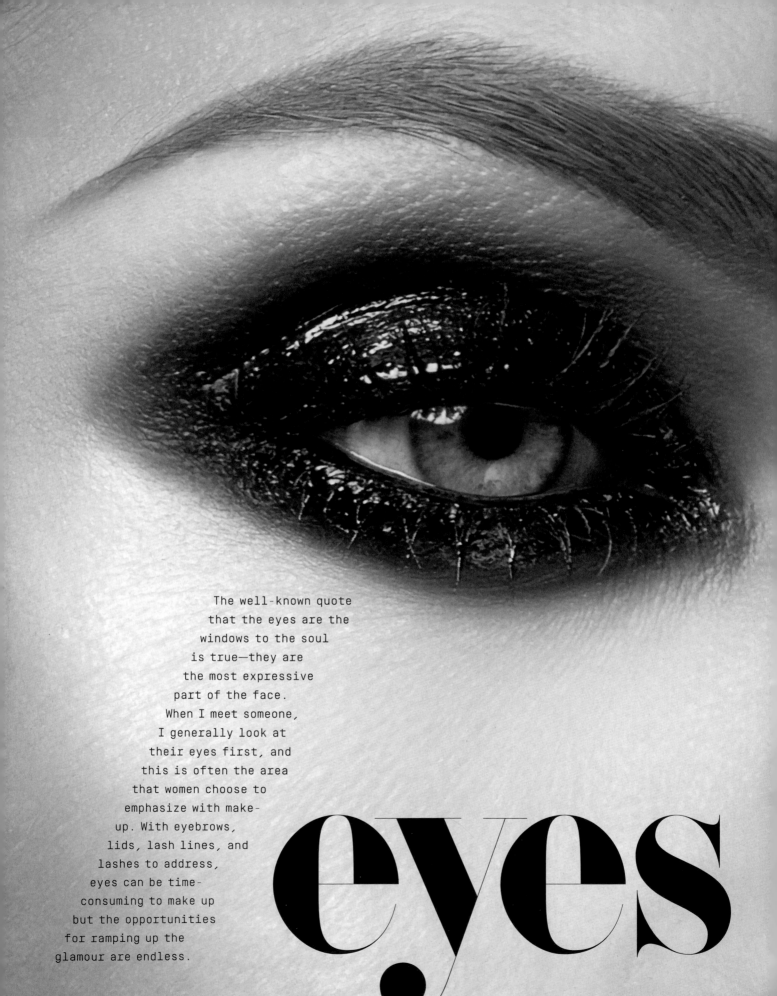

The well-known quote
that the eyes are the
windows to the soul
is true—they are
the most expressive
part of the face.
When I meet someone,
I generally look at
their eyes first, and
this is often the area
that women choose to
emphasize with make-
up. With eyebrows,
lids, lash lines, and
lashes to address,
eyes can be time-
consuming to make up
but the opportunities
for ramping up the
glamour are endless.

eyes

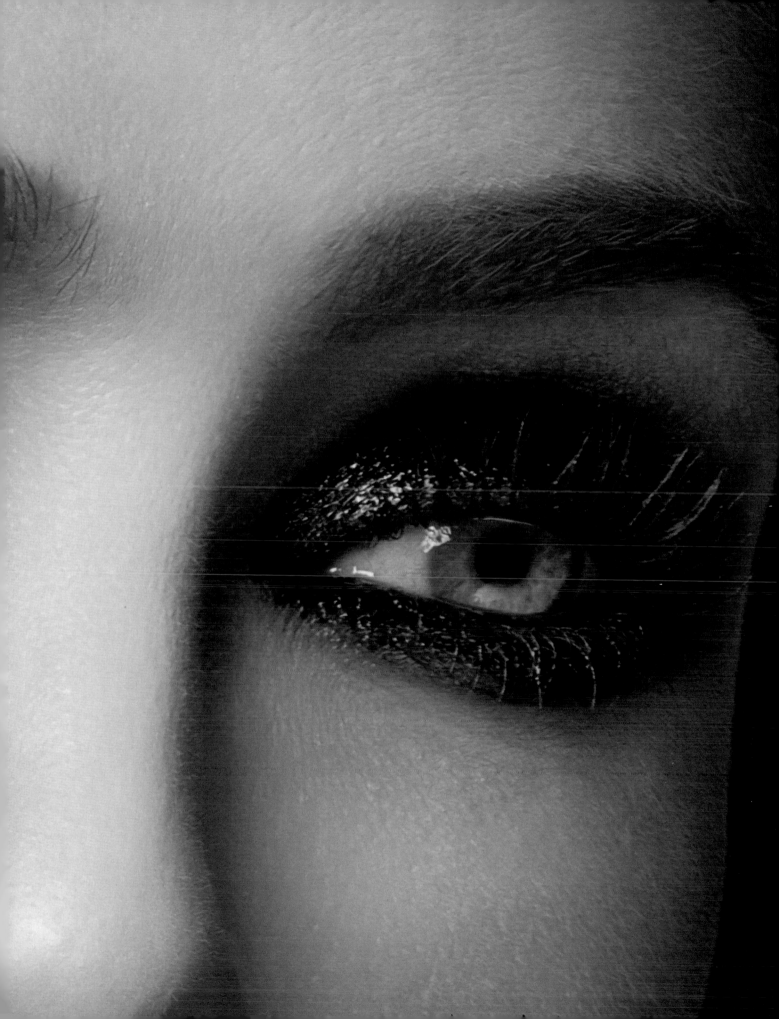

Eye 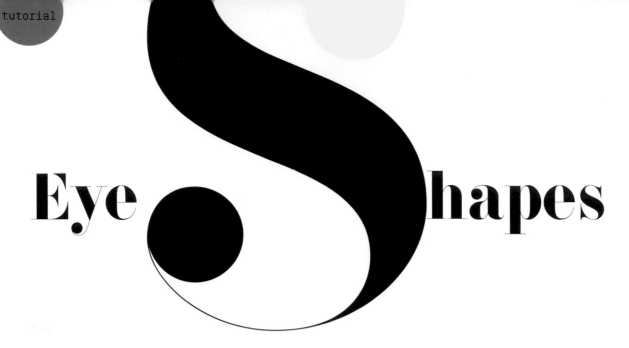 hapes

It's easy to underestimate the importance of determining your natural eye shape, forgetting just how far it affects what can be achieved when making up the eyes. The shape of the eyes dictates how they should be defined to bring out their best qualities—whether you should use eyeshadow or eyeliner, in what textures and tones, and where they should be applied to enhance your eyes. Everybody's eyes are different and it's always possible to create illusions if you know what it is that you're trying to improve and how to go about it.

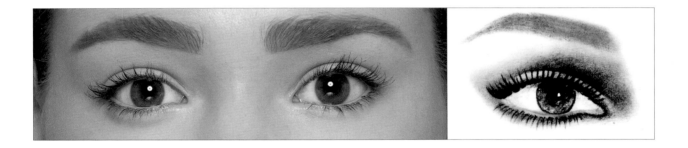

↑ **wide-set** To pull the eyes together, apply more depth at the beginning of the eyes and to the top and bottom lash lines. Taking the color as close to the tear ducts as possible, even onto the corner of the nose, draws the eyes closer together. Eyeliners and mascara can be taken all the way around the eyes to the inner corners.

↓ **close-set** If the eyes are too close together, it can make them look small and a bit cross-eyed. To counteract this, apply light eyeshadow at the inner corners of the eyes and add depth and darkness to the outer corners. Keep everything, including eyeliner and mascara, concentrated on the outer half of the eyes to draw them apart.

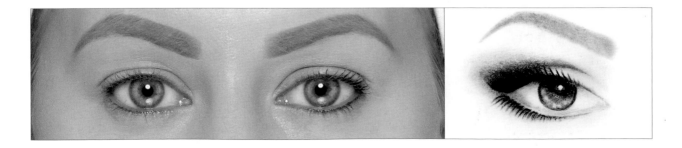

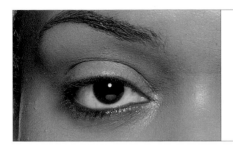
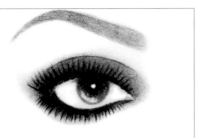

protruding Large lids can make the eyes look big and bulbous, so the aim is to minimize them by using darker tones with a matte finish, focusing on the middle part of the lids, so that everything is muted and doesn't shout for attention. Smoky eyes, eyeliner, and false lashes all look great, as they help disguise the size of the eyelids.

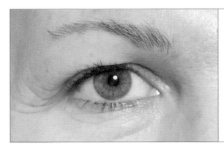
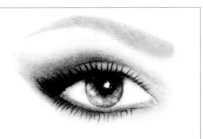

downturned/hooded To lift the eyes, use eyeliner to create a feline flick or blend eyeshadow into the socket, focusing on the outer two-thirds of the eye. For hooded eyes, apply dark eyeshadow above the socket, so you can see it when the eyes are open. Concentrate on defining the lash lines and lashes to make them the focus.

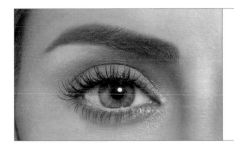
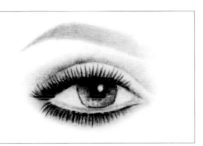

upturned/almond If you were born with this eye shape, you're lucky, as everything suits you, and the eyes naturally lift at the outer corners, giving you a fresh, wide-awake look. The lower lids can sometimes be as pronounced as the top lids, which means you can put eyeshadow under the eyes as well, for extra drama.

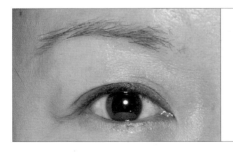
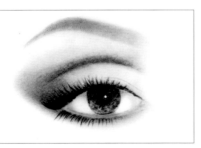

monolid This eye is quite flat with no socket, so the aim is to create a 3-D effect with graduating tones of eyeshadow. Keep dark colors close to the lash line, neutral tones in the middle, and light tones under the brow. See the steps on page 103 and the tips on page 104 for how to create a crease and make the eyes look bigger.

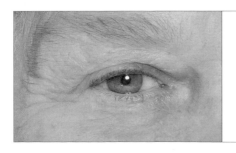
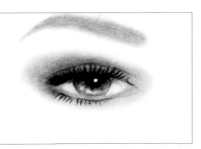

droopy Create a natural eyelift by curling the lashes and grooming the brows. Don't put mascara on your bottom lashes, as this will drag the eyes down, and avoid shimmery eyeshadows that will highlight wrinkles. Keep eyeliner as close to the roots as possible. A dark matte wash on the lids will add depth and make the eyes stand out.

Brows

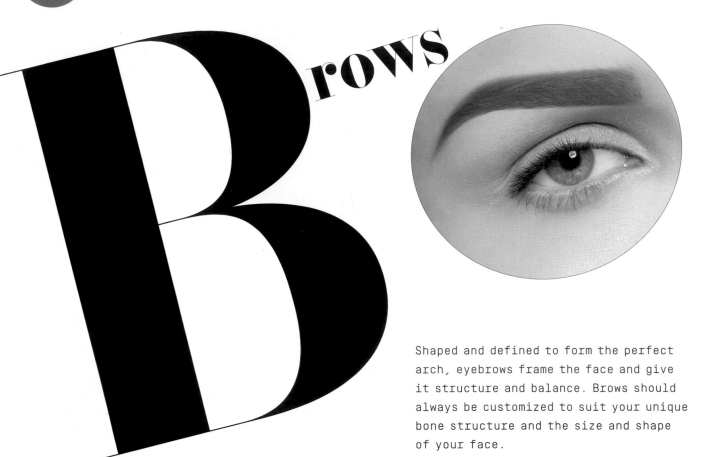

Shaped and defined to form the perfect arch, eyebrows frame the face and give it structure and balance. Brows should always be customized to suit your unique bone structure and the size and shape of your face.

Use the right-shaped tweezers for shaping your brows. I find it easier to grab the hairs if the tweezers have pointed or slanted tips. It's not true that you shouldn't pluck hairs from above your brows—just remember that the shaping that creates the arch and helps to "lift" the brow happens from underneath, and overplucking the top will push the brow down and create a straighter shape. If you have stubborn, unruly brows, brush them up and then trim them. To fill in sparse brows and correct the shape of the arch, use a pencil or a small angled brush and a matte powder, cream, clay, pomade, mousse, or gel. If you've got dark hair, go a shade lighter than your hair color. If you're blonde, go a shade darker. Ashy tones will look more natural than warm or red tones, unless you have red hair. For a natural look, keep your brows full and neat, brush them up and seal with a tinted gel.

Tips

» Don't do one brow and then try to match it; work on alternate eyes, plucking a couple of hairs from one and then the other, so you can match the shapes gradually.

» Don't overpluck the beginning of your brows, as it will make your nose look broader and your eyes too far apart.

» Don't make the high point of the arch too close to the middle of your brow, as it will make your eyes look narrow.

» Keep your brows as full as possible for a youthful appearance—making them too thin looks hard and aging, creates too much space, and makes your eyelids look puffy.

» If you are guilty of overplucking, be patient while they grow back and in the meantime fill in the shape with a brow powder or pencil.

» If you want to lighten or tattoo your brows, always get a professional to do it.

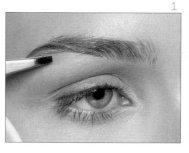
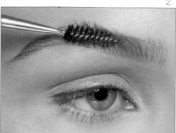
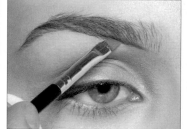
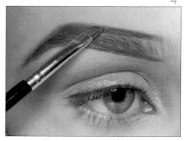

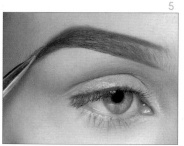
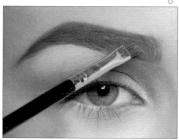
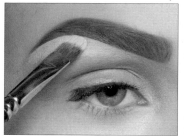
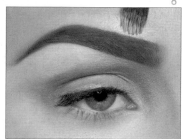

perfect contoured brows

For a glamorous, groomed look, the most flattering brows are slightly lighter at the beginning and gradually become more intense from the top of the arch to the tail.

1 Tweeze away any stray hairs to create a neat arch that suits your face shape and bone structure.

2 Brush the brows up and into their natural shape; you don't want to create a shape too far removed from this, as it will look unnatural.

3 Using a small angled brush and a brow powder or pomade, underline the brow. Do this precisely, without putting too much pressure on the brush, as the line should look quite soft, especially at the start of the eye.

4 In the same way, lightly outline the top, starting at the beginning of the brow and slanting the line up to where you've decided the highest point of the arch should be. If you want to create a fuller brow, take the line very slightly above the natural hairline.

5 Take the line down the outer tail from the top of the arch to the tip, just beyond the outer corner of the eye.

6 Using what's left of the product on your brush, fill in any gaps with light, feathery strokes, concentrating the depth of color on the mid-section and arch.

7 To create a really dynamic brow, apply a little concealer or foundation underneath the brow to keep the line clean. Using a shade slightly lighter than your skin tone really draws attention to the brows.

8 Do the same above your brows to emphasize the shape and make your eyebrows look really precise.

SQUARE FACES look better with a soft, rounder brow shape.

ROUND FACES look better with a slightly higher arch.

LONG FACES look better with an extended brow.

OVAL AND HEART-SHAPED FACES look better with a gentle arch.

creating the perfect shape

The key to creating a gorgeous brow is to imagine that it's divided into thirds. The thickest end should start just beyond the bridge of the nose; the highest point of the arch should be just beyond the outside edge of the pupil; and the thinnest end should finish just beyond the outer corner. An easy way to create the perfect shape is to take the thinnest make-up brush you have and hold it at an angle at the corner of your nose so it lines up with the outer edge of your pupil. The point where the brush crosses your brow is where the highest part of the arch should be.

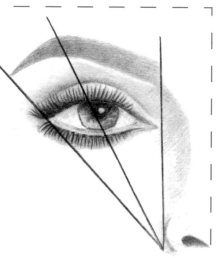

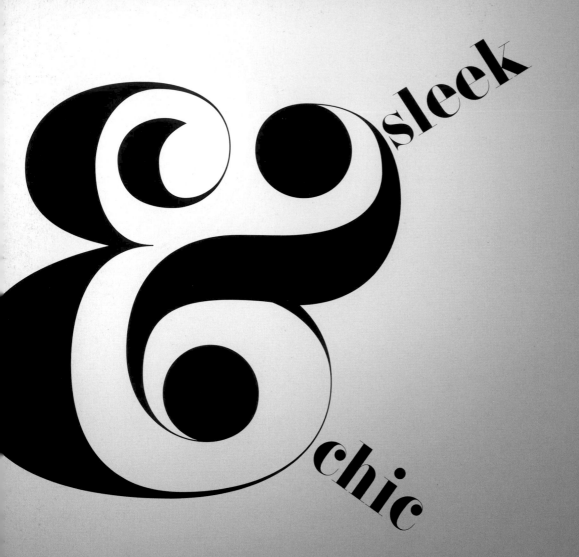

& sleek

chic

This is grown-up, sophisticated make-up, with the focus on defining the eyes in an understated way for everyday glamour.

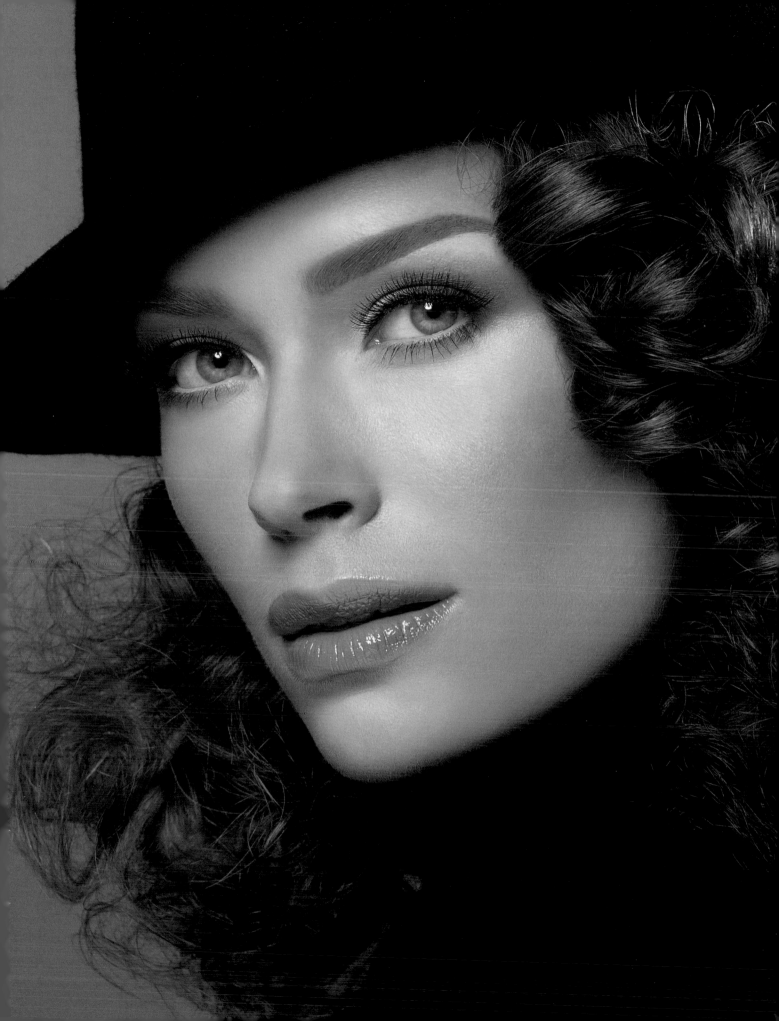

Sleek and Chic Transformation

The look is beautiful and refined in a low-key way, with wearable make-up that is perfect for any daytime occasion, from a wedding to work. The skin looks radiant, the eyes are defined in a classic, understated way and the lips are enhanced with creamy, nude lipstick for a luxurious finish. The textures of the make-up are soft and matte, while the colors are warm and flattering to the skin tone, with nothing to make a statement or create too much drama. Our model [previous spread] has fair skin with pink undertones, so I selected soft, pink-based shades of taupe and brown to enhance her eyes, rose-petal blush and beige-pink lipstick.

For the transformation on Leena, I chose eyeshadows in deeper, orange-based nude and brown shades, apricot blush and peachy-pink, café-au-lait lipstick to flatter her skin tone. I find that Asian women often make their lips the focus of their look, using just eyeliner and mascara on their eyes, and I wanted to show an accessible way to contour the eyes to make them look larger and more open. Leena's eyes are long and narrow, with small eyelids and shallow creases, so my aim was to create depth above the natural sockets to give the illusion of more space on the lids. This makes her eyes look rounder and beautifully defined.

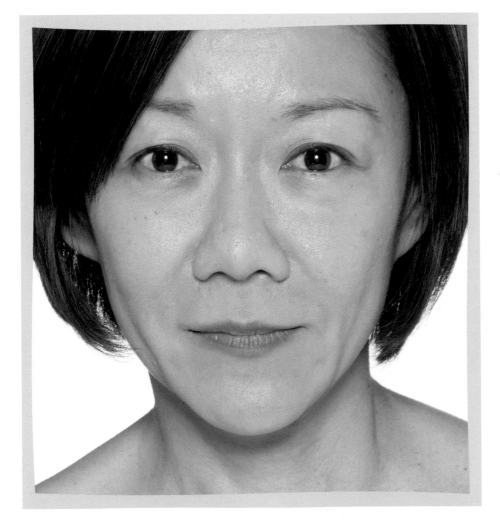

Leena is a great-looking lady in her forties, who wanted to know how to make the best of her face. In particular, she wanted to learn how to make her eyes look bigger and create more of a socket.

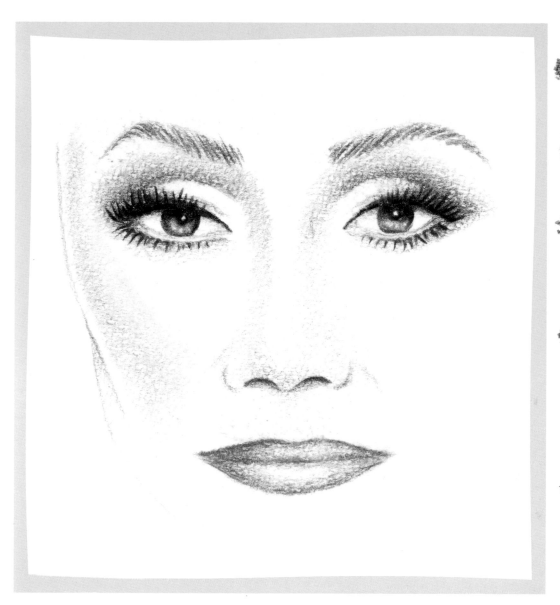

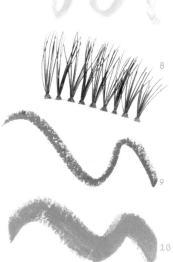

face

Anti-aging, collagen-
boosting primer.
Liquid foundation to
match the skin tone.
Light and dark shades
of cream foundation and
powder for contouring.
Warm, soft, brick-colored
blush (1).
Highlighter.

eyes

Soft brown matte brow powder.
Brow gel.
Bone-colored matte powder
eyeshadow (2).
Mid-brown matte powder
eyeshadow with a reddish
undertone (3).
Dark chocolate-brown matte
powder eyeshadow (4).
Slightly shimmery
highlighter (5).
Black gel eyeliner (6).
Nude eyeliner pencil (7).
Black mascara.
Three-quarter lashes (8).

lips

Flesh-toned, pinky brown
lip liner (9).
Slightly lighter lipstick
in the same tone (10).

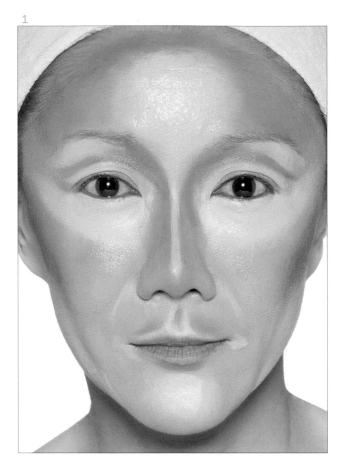

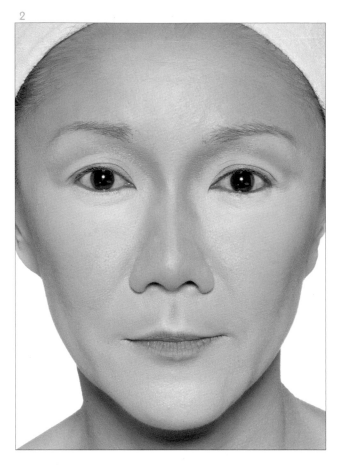

■face

1 After cleansing the face, tidying the brows, and applying anti-aging, collagen-boosting primer, I chose a liquid foundation to match her skin tone and create a good base.

Leena has a slim, heart-shaped face, so I needed to contour it only lightly to bring out her cheekbones and slim down her nose, using light and dark shades of cream foundation and powder (see pages 56–61). Because she has a very slim jaw, I didn't take the darker shade any lower than the base of her nose, but I did use it to begin to contour her eyes, drawing on an imaginary socket line that I later built on with eyeshadow to give it further definition.

2 I blended the contouring creams with a soft blending brush for a flawless finish and then warmed up her cheeks with a soft, brick-colored blush on the apples. I also applied a touch of highlighter on the apples of her cheeks and above her upper lip to catch the light and make her face look softer and fuller.

Tip To work out where to draw your new socket crease, look straight ahead in a mirror and follow the shape of your natural socket line but draw the new one a fraction above it, using either pencil or eyeshadow.

3

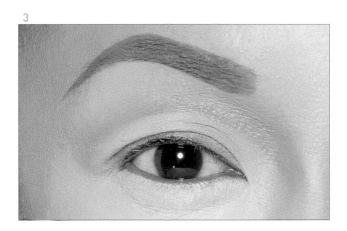

4

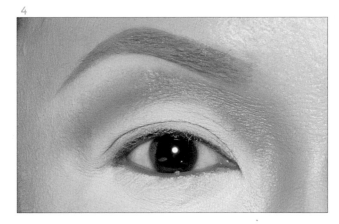

5

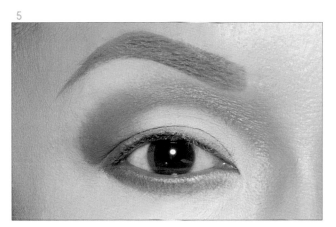

6

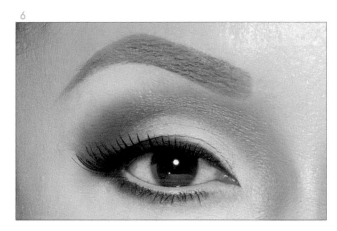

▪ eyes

3 I wanted to give her more of an arch to lift the eyebrows, so I built up the shape using a small angled brush and matte brow powder in a soft brown. Once I'd created the shape I wanted, I sealed the brows with brow gel to keep them in place.

4 First, I applied a bone-colored matte eyeshadow over the entire eye area, from the lash line to the brow bone, with a medium eyeshadow brush. Then, with a small angled brush, I sketched in a new socket crease over the earlier contouring using a matte eyeshadow in a mid-brown with a red undertone.

5 At the outer corner of the eye, I drew a line down from the new socket crease to the lash line, just below the arch of the brow, and blended the eyeshadow into the outer V-shaped corner of the eye between the crease and the lash line. Then, with a round pencil brush, I swept the same color underneath the lower lash line. This has the effect of lifting the eyes, creating the illusion of space on the eyelid and adding drama and depth using tone and shadow.

6 This look is all about definition, so once I'd created the shape and crease I wanted, I intensified it with a dark chocolate-brown matte eyeshadow, blended into the outer corners of the eyes to draw them further apart and into the creases to give them definition and depth, which makes the eyes look bigger and lifted.

I then added a slightly shimmery highlighter under the brow bone and a little in the middle of the lid; this light sheen draws the eye to give the illusion of more space and dimension, as well as softening the matte look.

Using a small angled brush, I applied a black gel eyeliner to the upper lash line, thickening and lifting the line from just beyond the center toward the outer corners of the eyes (see pages 148–9). I went over this line with the dark chocolate-brown matte eyeshadow, which I also took under the lower lashes at the outer corners.

To brighten and open up the eyes, I applied a nude eyeliner pencil along the lower waterline.

I curled the lashes and applied a coat of black mascara. Then I added three-quarter lashes to the outer edges of the eyes, which lifts them at the outer corners (see page 137). I coated the lower lashes with mascara and then added a little more to the roots of the upper lashes for extra volume and to blend her natural lashes with the false ones.

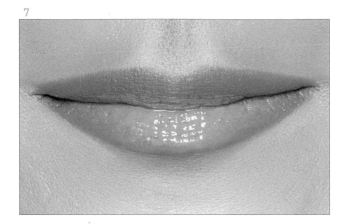

7

■lips

7 I primed the lips with foundation to neutralize their natural pigment, as I wanted to create soft, nude-brown lips. I chose a flesh-toned, pinky brown lip liner and lipstick to complement the colors used on her face and eyes, so all the tones worked together for a neutral finish. I outlined the lips first, to perfect the shape, and blotted and reapplied, and then did the same with the lipstick for a classic, beautiful finish.

Tips

» This is an elegant, polished look, so make sure you are well-groomed from top to toe.

» Hair should be freshly washed and blow-dried in a timeless style that works well with the make-up.

» Have your nails manicured and painted in a nude shade to suit your skin tone.

» Choose clothes that are chic and understated, in neutral tones and classic cuts, to bring the whole look together.

» Try a stronger shade of lipstick to suit your skin tone. With the eyes played down in neutrals, you can afford a brighter lip color, which exudes confidence.

how to make your eyes look bigger

» Medical-grade eyelid tape and glue are really popular ways to create a new crease or to even out uneven eyelids. You need to identify where you want your new crease to be, apply the tape or glue and use an eyelid prong to gently push the lid into place. This technique can be used to create a higher socket that makes the eye look bigger.

» Wearing colored contact lenses with a diameter greater than the iris makes the eyes look much larger than they are.

» Always curl your lashes to open up the eyes; you can also have them permed.

» Invest in some false lashes, which make the eyes look bigger and more defined.

» Creating a great arch shape for your eyebrows will give your eyes a wide-awake look.

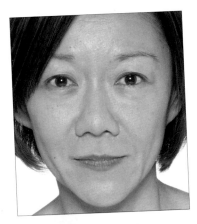

"I'm a full-time mother of two teenage girls, and home life is pretty full-on and busy with the kids, so it was a real treat and a fantastic experience to be completely made over by such a talented artist as Gary—and to turn out looking so fabulous was amazing."

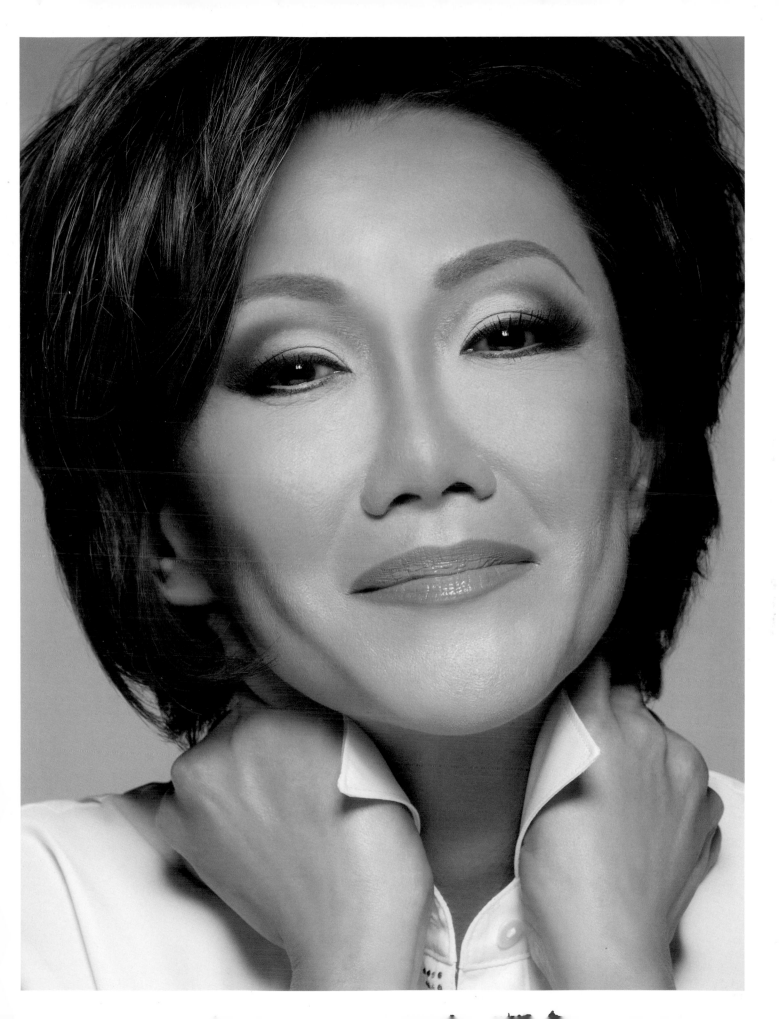

Eye textures and finishes

What would we do without all that wonderful choice of eyeshadow, with its vast array of tones, textures, and finishes that give us such an easy way to add color and drama to a look? The style of your eye make-up dictates your entire look, whether it's soft and natural or more intense, matte or glossy, full-on or an accent. Eyeshadow gives you the opportunity to create endless visual delights—there really are no limits to what you can do.

Powder eyeshadows can be pressed or loose. They are easy to apply and blend and can be layered with other textures, such as cream or glitter. Cream eyeshadows come in either a palette or tube, or in a pencil or crayon format. Creams tend to give a high-shine finish but are prone to creasing, making them high-maintenance and not so long-lasting as most powder eyeshadows. I usually apply powder eyeshadow with a natural-bristle brush and cream ones with a synthetic brush.

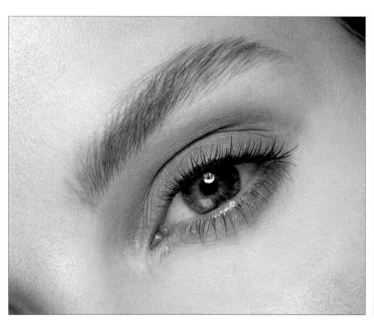 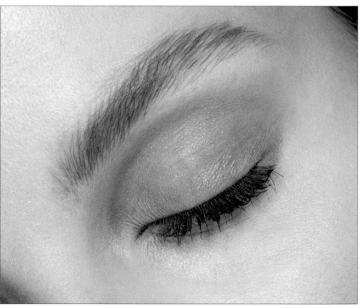

sheer

If you have only minutes in your day to apply some sort of look to your eye, sheer eyeshadow is the perfect choice. It's simple, wearable, low-maintenance, and great for the daytime. The most obvious look to create is a barely-there wash of color—whether a neutral tone or light, pastel shade. Sheer eyeshadows look great on women of any age, as the effect is soft and subtle. They can be either cream or powder, matte or shimmer, and are very easy to build up to achieve the desired effect. Many sheer products are multipurpose and so work on the eyes, cheeks, and lips, which saves money and time.

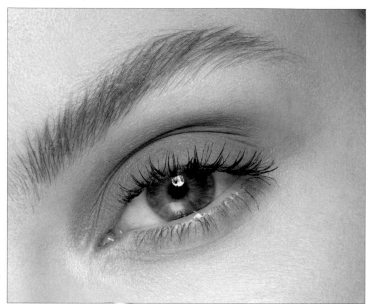

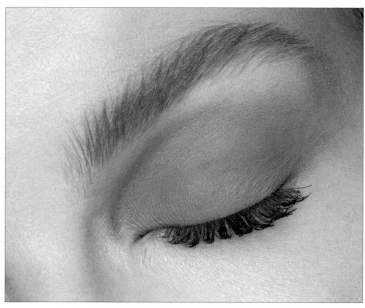

matte

Flat, matte eyeshadow comes in a cream format but is more often a pressed powder with no light-reflective particles, so it absorbs the light, drawing in the color and providing more depth. It can look very subtle in neutral tones or more dramatic in darker colors, with a finish that always reminds me of velvet. Using a primer first helps to intensify the color and makes it last longer. Matte eyeshadow looks good on more mature eyes, as it flattens out fine lines and doesn't draw attention to them as a shimmer would. It is also ideal for cutting out a crease and creating depth and definition, and can be combined with shimmer shadows to great effect.

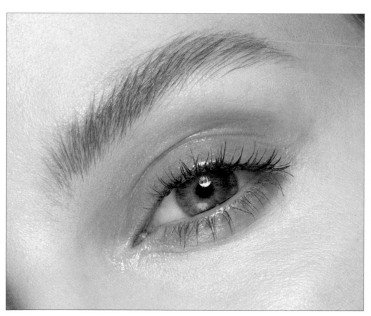

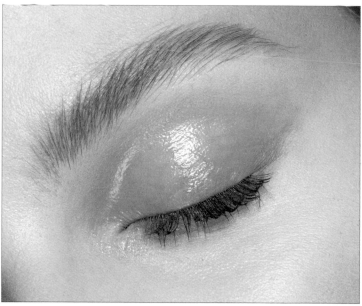

gloss

I love the watery look that gloss gives to the eyes and I often use petroleum jelly or Eight Hour Cream to achieve this. It can be applied to bare eyelids for a sheer, ethereal effect, be layered over a color to give it a glazed, lacquered finish, or be added to a smoky eye for an edgy, urban look. You can also buy gloss eyeshadows that contain color pigment. It's the hardest eye texture to apply and wear, as it tends to travel, so be prepared to touch it up. A little goes a long way, so take your time applying it, dabbing it on with your finger or a small flat brush. Used as an accent on the beginning of your eye or under your waterline, it changes your look in an instant.

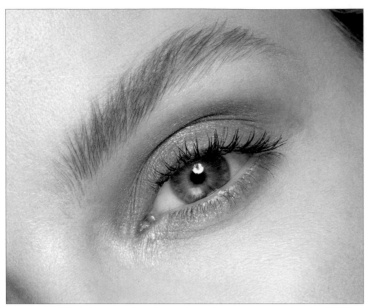
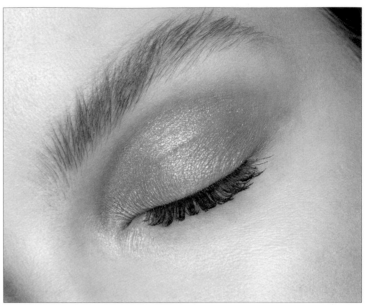

shimmer

This is possibly the most popular eyeshadow to wear, as a little shimmer on the lids brings the eyes alive and makes the skin look radiant. Shimmer eyeshadow has a light-reflective finish but the sheen is subtle, so it can be worn in the day or evening, and you can incorporate it with other textures to build up a dramatic look. It's easy to apply and blend, and it looks great all over the eye or subtly applied under the brow bone or on the beginning of the eyes. Shimmer will highlight fine lines, so as you get older, keep it to the taut area of the eyes, usually the mid-section of the lid, and avoid the brow bone or anywhere that wrinkles when you smile.

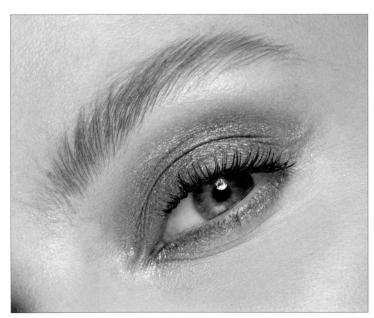
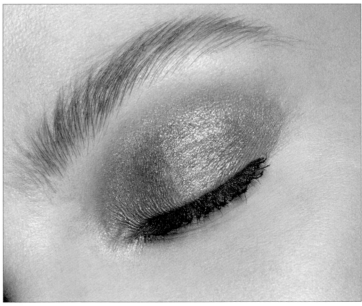

pigment

A loose-powder eyeshadow with a high concentration of color and light-reflective properties, pigment can be used to add drama and intensity to a look, as well as giving a high-shine finish. The color is long-lasting and vivid and pigment is very easy to blend, but you need only a little, so apply it gradually. Vibrantly colored or metallic pigments can be used as highlighters, or you can mix them into different mediums, such as lip glosses and lotions. If you're not brave enough to try a glossy texture on your eyes, pigment is your next best option, as you can build it up to achieve that high-shine, liquid look.

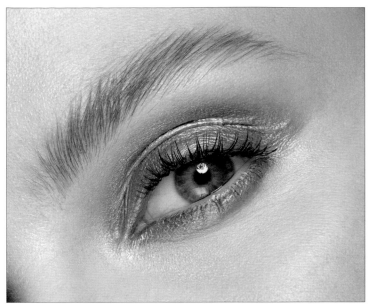 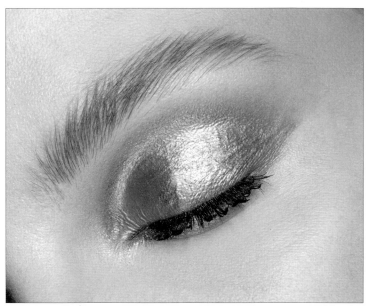

metallic

For a rich, opulent look, nothing beats a metallic eyeshadow, which gives the eyes a luscious sheen. It produces quite an intense result, but it can also be used as an accent for highlighting areas such as the beginning of the eye, the lash line, or the mid-section of the lid. Choose a shade that suits your skin tone: silver and platinum tend to look good on fair skin, while bronze and gold suit olive and dark skin tones; rose gold works on everybody. Metallics comes in a variety of textures—cream and powder eyeshadows as well as eyeliners. As with all light-reflective products, be careful not to apply it on areas where it will draw attention to fine lines.

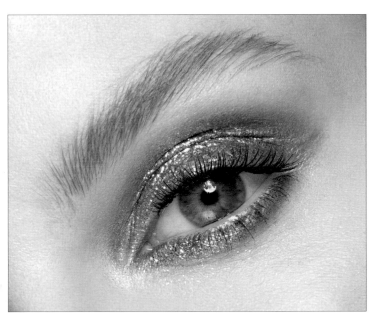 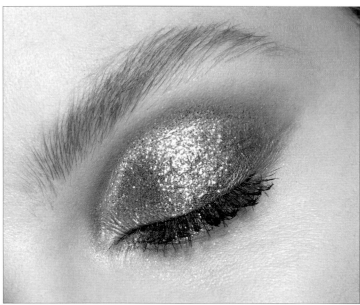

glitter

If you want to glam the whole thing up and take the eyes to the max, try glitter—it's a great way to dress eyes up for the evening. These small, light-reflective, sparkly particles usually need a cream base in order for them to stick to the skin. Eye glitter comes in different grades in an array of colors, from vibrant to metallic. Finer particles will give a subtle finish and are best if you have small eyes; larger particles are more flamboyant and showy but can look very striking—just be careful that they don't settle into lines and make the eyes look heavy. Getting the right balance takes practice, but you can have lots of fun with glitter—and that's what it's all about.

Smoking hot

The smoky eye is one of the most iconic make-up looks that I'm always asked to create. It's the ultimate sexy eye.

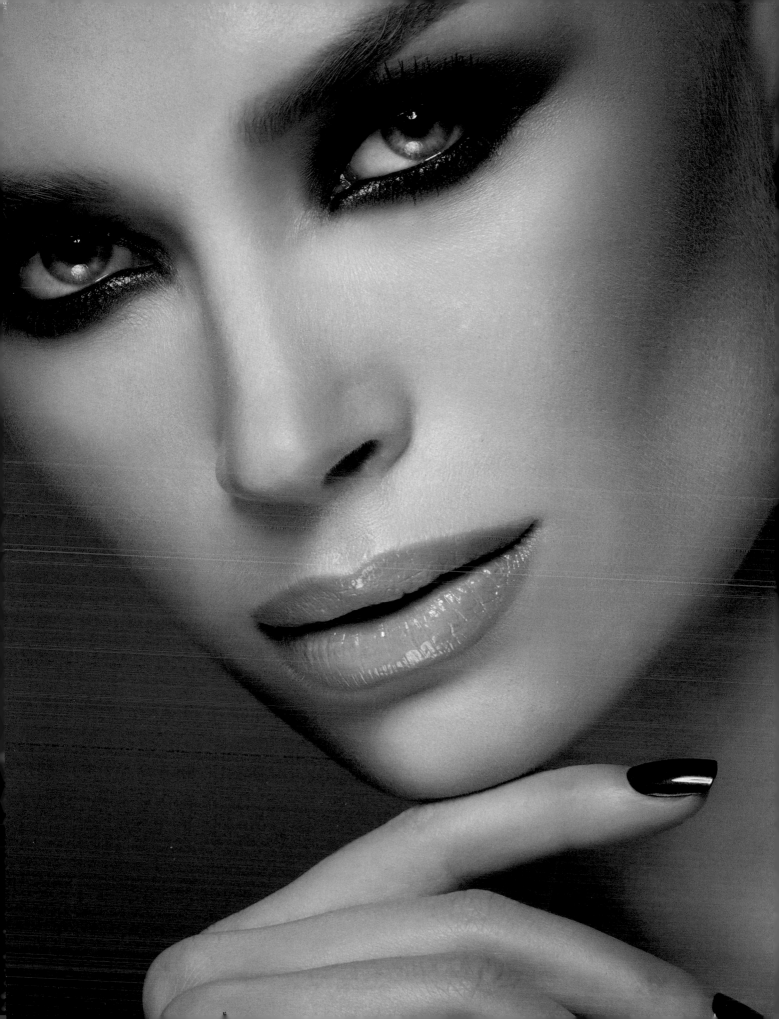

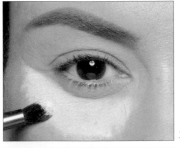

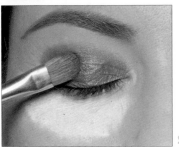

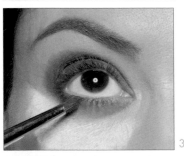

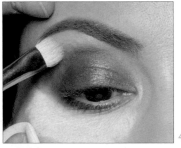

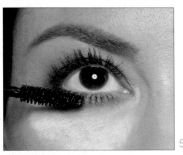

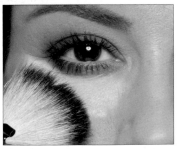

Sultry Smoky Eye

With her stunning, exotic looks, television presenter Melanie Sykes has the most beautiful eyes to demonstrate how versatile this look can be, as all the examples look fantastic on her. Opposite is an everyday smoky eye that is quick to achieve with a simple wash of eyeshadow. You can use any color, but chocolates and taupes suit everyone and always look sophisticated. The result is a full lid of texture and tone with soft, smoky edges. It's the lightest smoky eye and works well for daytime. Marry it with natural brows, a dewy, liquid foundation, and light contouring, if you need it, with warm apricot blush and pinkish nude lipstick.

1 As I'd already made up her face, I brushed a layer of translucent powder under her eyes in case any eyeshadow dropped onto her cheeks.

2 I chose a mushroomy mid-brown eyeshadow with a soft shimmer. Shimmer eyeshadow blends more easily than matte and, because it reflects light, it tends to look softer on the eye. I used a medium eyeshadow brush to apply it over the whole of the eyelid and gently blended it upward over the crease and outward to the outer corner of the eye.

3 With a pencil brush, I took the eyeshadow underneath the eye from the outer corner, softening it from the mid-point toward the inner corner and blending it to nothing.

4 A smoky eye is all about the blending, so I used a fluffy brush to soften any hard lines all around the outer edge of the eyeshadow.

5 I curled the lashes to create a wide-open eye and then applied black mascara to the top and bottom lashes.

6 Once the lashes were dry, I used a fan-shaped brush to thoroughly brush away the powder under the eyes.

smoky eye tool kit

You can get away with three or four brushes for this look:

Flat mid-sized brush for applying the eyeshadow to the lid.

Small round pencil brush or angled brush for taking the color under the eye.

Soft, fluffy blending brush for blending—press the brush gently against the back of your hand and if the bristles fan out, it's perfect for the job.

Synthetic brush for helping to push the powder into the skin. It is also good for layering on textures to create added intensity.

Tip Think of black mascara as the "little black dress" of make-up. How much you put on is a personal thing—it depends on what suits you, what you feel comfortable with, and the occasion.

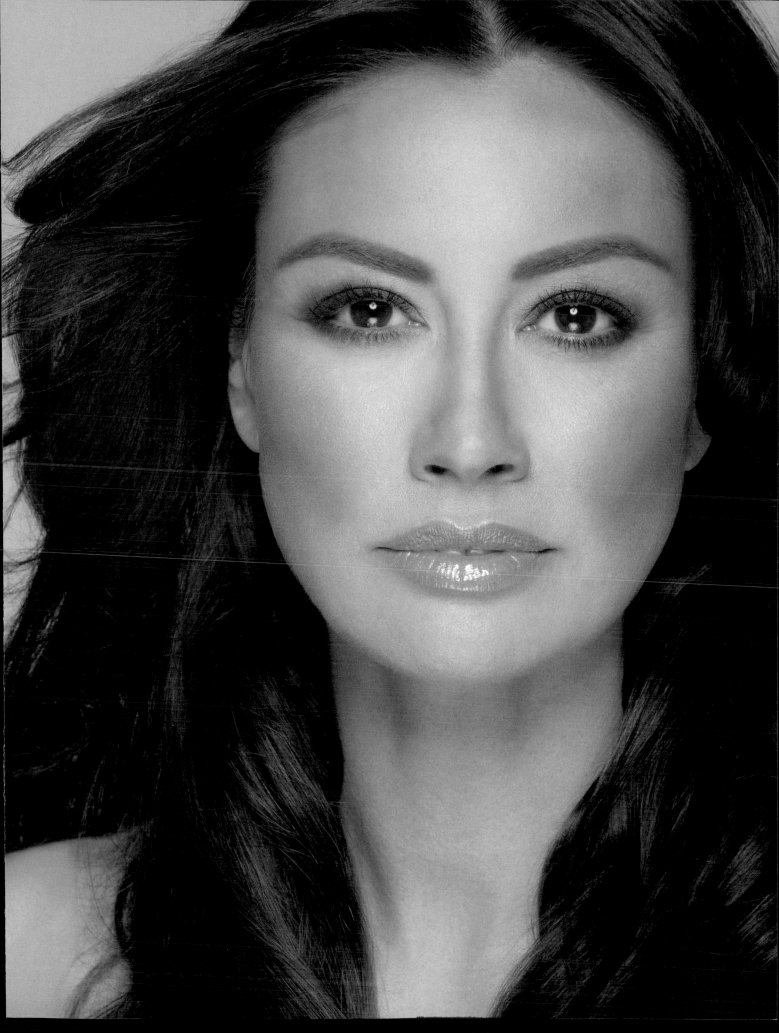

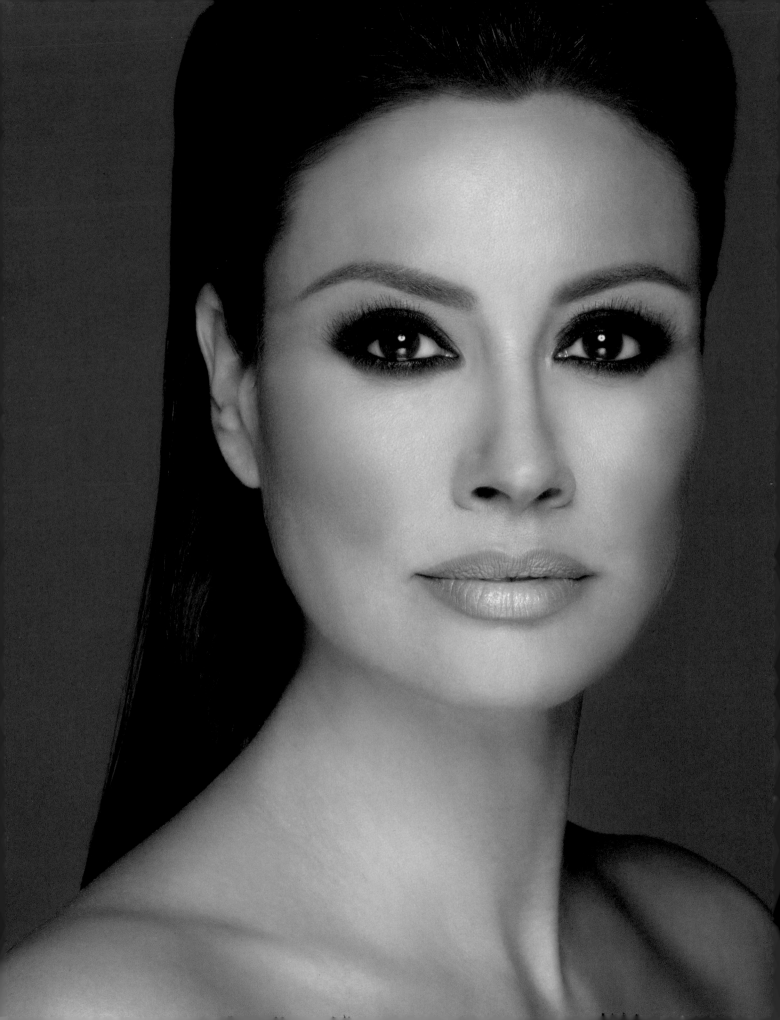

Bedroom Eyes

This is the most popular smoky eye that everyone wants to learn how to achieve. For this classic interpretation on Melanie, who epitomizes glamour, I chose charcoal tones to create drama and depth, but I built on top of the mushroom-brown wash I had already done, as the warm undertone softens the gray and makes it sit better on the skin. A matte eyeshadow is key, as the finish should look like velvet. This sexy eye is complemented by velvety matte foundation with subtle contouring and a luxurious, creamy satin lipstick in a soft caramel.

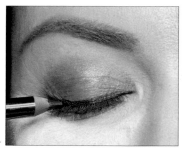

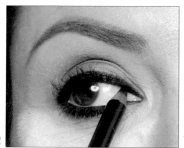

keep it clean

Dark, powdery textures will definitely have fallout, but there are ways to combat this ultimate black-eye disaster:

» My favorite old trick is to apply translucent powder under the eyes, so that if any eyeshadow falls on the skin, you can sweep it away. When you are older, powder will settle in wrinkles and draw attention to them, so make sure you polish the skin well with your brush to remove it all.

» Shadow shields are pieces of sticky-back plastic that you put over the skin underneath your eyes.

» You can also hold a tissue under your eye—this is a useful trick as you can angle it as necessary.

» If you're not confident, do your smoky eye before the rest of your make-up.

Tips

» How low to blend color under the eyes depends on the eye shape. If your eyes are long, take the color lower to make them look rounder; if your eyes are round, take the line further out to elongate them.

» Dipping your brush into a little translucent powder makes blending easier.

1 After applying translucent powder under the eyes to protect the make-up, I lined the entire eye with a creamy black kohl pencil, starting at the beginning of the upper lash line and then taking it under the eye and inside the waterline.

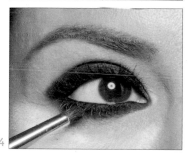

2 I went around the eye a few times to thicken the line and increase the depth. The aim is for all the intensity and drama to start at the roots of the lashes and then, as everything is blended outward, it becomes softer and softer.

3 I applied a rich, dark, smoky brown eyeshadow with a semi-matte finish all over the lid, blending it up and inward from the outer edge to create depth, and softening it outward at the crease.

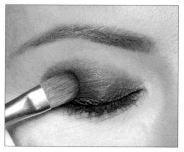

4 With a small pencil brush, I swept the same eyeshadow under the eye and blended it well, to soften the line to a smoky finish.

5 I took a soft-bristled brush and blended everything again, working in small, circular motions all around the eye to soften any hard edges.

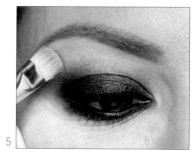

6 After curling the upper lashes and applying a fine coat of black mascara to the top and bottom lashes, I added clusters of false lashes to the outer edge of the eye, stopping midway. This creates a fluttery doe eye that still looks really natural. I finished the eyes with another coat of mascara on the top lashes and, when it was dry, I brushed the translucent powder off her cheeks.

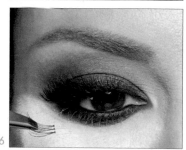

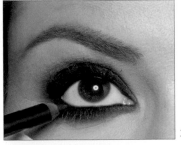

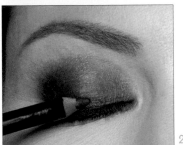

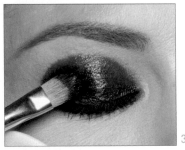

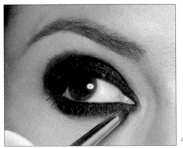

Rock-Chick Eyes

Only for the brave—and carried off to perfection by Melanie—
this shiny, slightly messy smoky eye is the hardest to wear, as the
greasy finish is high-maintenance and prone to creasing, but if you
get it right, it can be really sexy. It's an edgy look that isn't
about perfection; make it as messed-up as you like, but try it at
home before you wear it out, as these textures have a tendency to
slide around. Matte foundation would look wrong with the high-shine
eyes, so I applied a luminous, dewy foundation, a creamy blush for
a natural-looking flush, and a pinky nude lip gloss.

1 To intensify the previous
look and take it to the next level,
I really went to town with the kohl
eyeliner pencil, applying it around
the eye and inside the waterline.

2 I then took the pencil up from
the lash line onto the eyelid to
add a creamy texture. This may
be enough for you, but if not, go
to the next step.

3 Using a synthetic brush,
I applied petroleum jelly to the
eyelid, following its natural shape.

4 I used a small brush to add
a smear of petroleum jelly to the
inner corner of the eye, followed
by lashings of mascara—the
clumpier the better.

smoky eye top tips

» There's no eye shape that won't
  suit a smoky eye.

» There is no set color scheme—a
  smoky eye is all about the finish.

» Soft brown, taupe, and bronze tones
  are perfect for daytime smoky eyes.

» Stay away from flat blues and
  grays, which can make the eyes
  look dull and the skin sallow.
  A warm undertone and a slight
  shimmer will add warmth and light.

» This is a fantastic look if
  your lips aren't your strongest
  feature, as all the attention
  is drawn to the eyes.

» Always apply an eye primer to
  create a good base for the eye
  make-up—if an eyelid is too oily,
  it can make the eyeshadow break up.

» For extra drama and depth, use a
  primer, cream eyeshadow, or crayon
  on the lid first and apply the dark
  eyeshadow on top. This base helps
  prevent fallout and makes the eye
  make-up last longer, as it gives
  the powder something to stick to
  and intensifies its color.

» A creamy pencil liner that is easy
  to smudge is better for this look
  than gel liner, which gives a more
  precise line.

You can fake a wet-look smoky eye
with a high-shimmer pigment.
This gives the impression of a shimmery,
watery eye but lasts a lot longer.

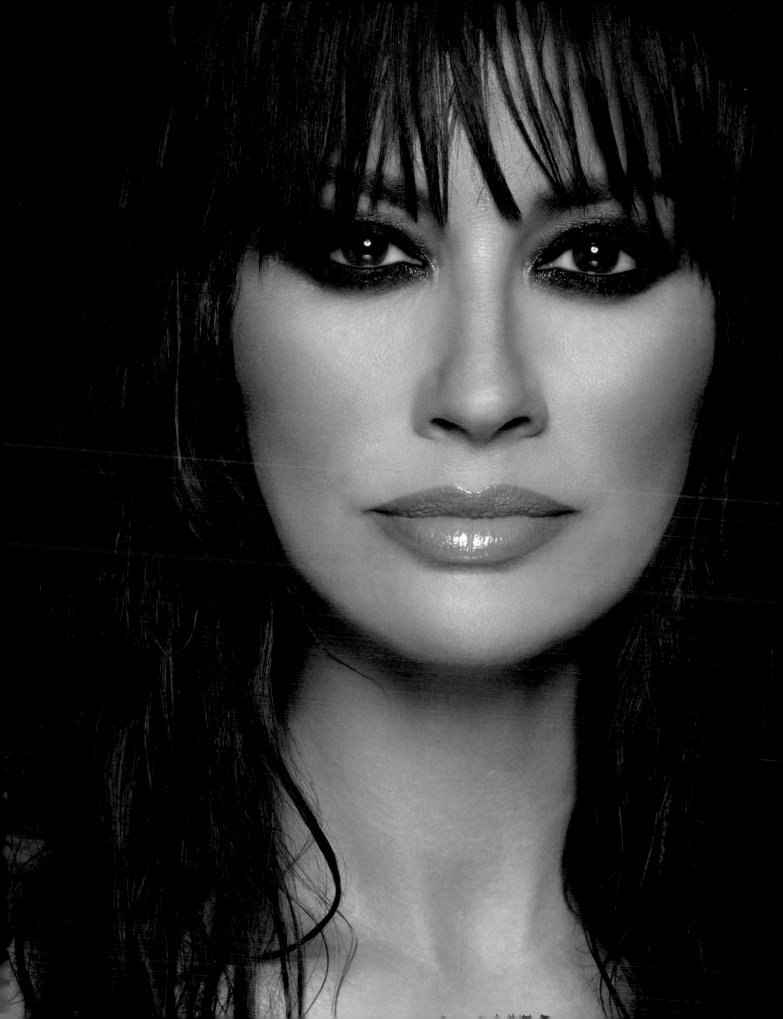

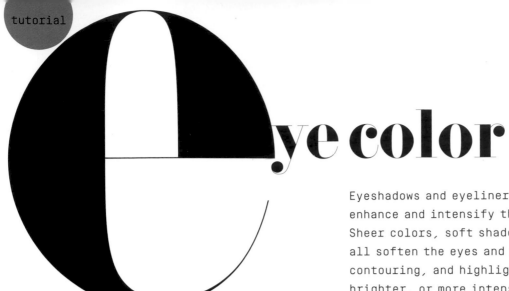

Eye color

Eyeshadows and eyeliners can dramatically enhance and intensify the color of your eyes. Sheer colors, soft shades, neutrals, and nudes all soften the eyes and are great for shading, contouring, and highlighting the eyes. Darker, brighter, or more intense colors make the eyes pop and help to create shape and depth.

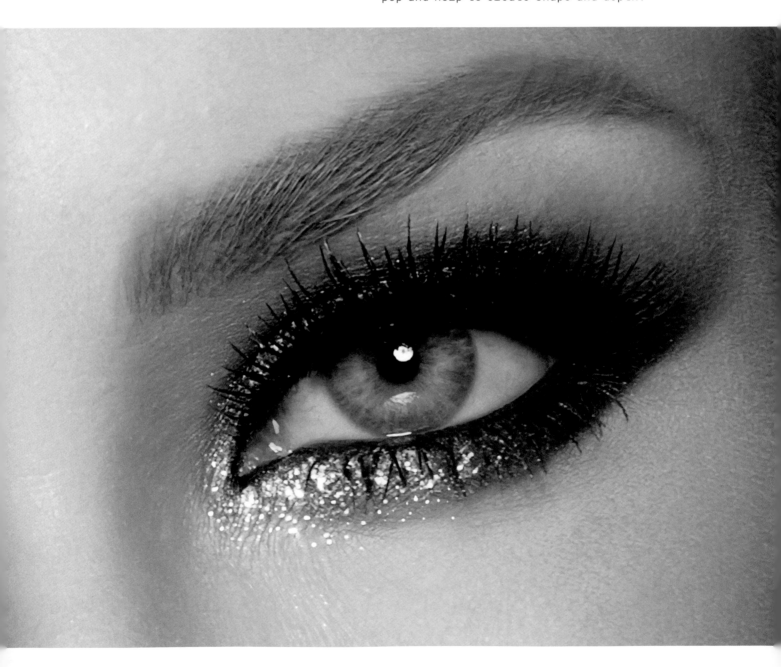

I didn't go to make-up school and I'm totally self-taught, so what I've learned about color began when I was a child, drawing on paper with colored crayons and knowing in my mind what I thought worked. Now, I can look at a person—their face, eyes, hair—and know instinctively what colors will make them look beautiful and glamorous. For me, it's about creating a mood and a look that makes the person feel and look wonderful.

Anyone can wear color, at any age—it's about finding out what shades suit you and what techniques and types of application work best for your eyes. There are textbook guidelines you can follow, such as the principle of the color wheel, which suggests choosing a color directly opposite the one that most closely matches your eye color. This can be a good starting point, but I think make-up should be fun and about expressing your individuality, so be brave with color and start experimenting. What works for one person may not work for another and you'll soon know when you put it on whether you like it—if you don't, just wash it off and start again. Rules should sometimes be broken, and what you think won't suit you might actually look amazing.

A simple way to start is with a good base shadow, which is usually applied to the mid-section of the lid. Next, you need a complementary darker tone for defining the outer edge of the eye and for contouring the socket, and a lighter tone to highlight the beginning of the eye and under the brow bone to lift and brighten the eye. Then, if you wish, you can use accent colors, pigments, or glitters to make the eyes pop. By adding pigment and combining different eyeshadow textures, you can create really dynamic looks, while jewel tones used as accents add that extra bit of glamour and really bring the eyes alive.

how to choose colors

Skin tone, hair, and eye color should all be taken into account when you're choosing a color for your eyes. Don't try to match your eyeshadow with the color of your eyes, as this tends to dull down the effect and can make you look too "pantomime-ready;" if you want to use the same color, go for a slightly different shade and use it as an accent. Here are some suggestions to try:

eye color

brown eyes Coppers, ambers, grays, charcoals, purples, greens, peaches, bronzes, teals, navy

blue/gray eyes Peaches, purples, silvers, pink tones, oranges, coppers, bronzes, golds, slate

green eyes Burgundies, berry tones, purples, rusts, mauves, plums, apricots, grays

hazel eyes Purples, rich golds, yellowy browns, dusty pinks, grays, taupes

skin tone

light Silver hues, subtle washes, soft tones

fair Taupes, browns, golds, soft tones

medium Greens, plums, purples, golds, bronzes

dark Red tones, taupes, bronzes, golds, purples

deep The most pigmented colors, rich purples, deep red-based tones, nothing ashy or too pearlized

hair color

brunette Browns, golds, greens, purples, black

blonde Golds, pinks, grays, black, greens, blues

red Pinks, golds, greens, olives, black

Navy looks great with any eye color
and is a good substitute for black.

119

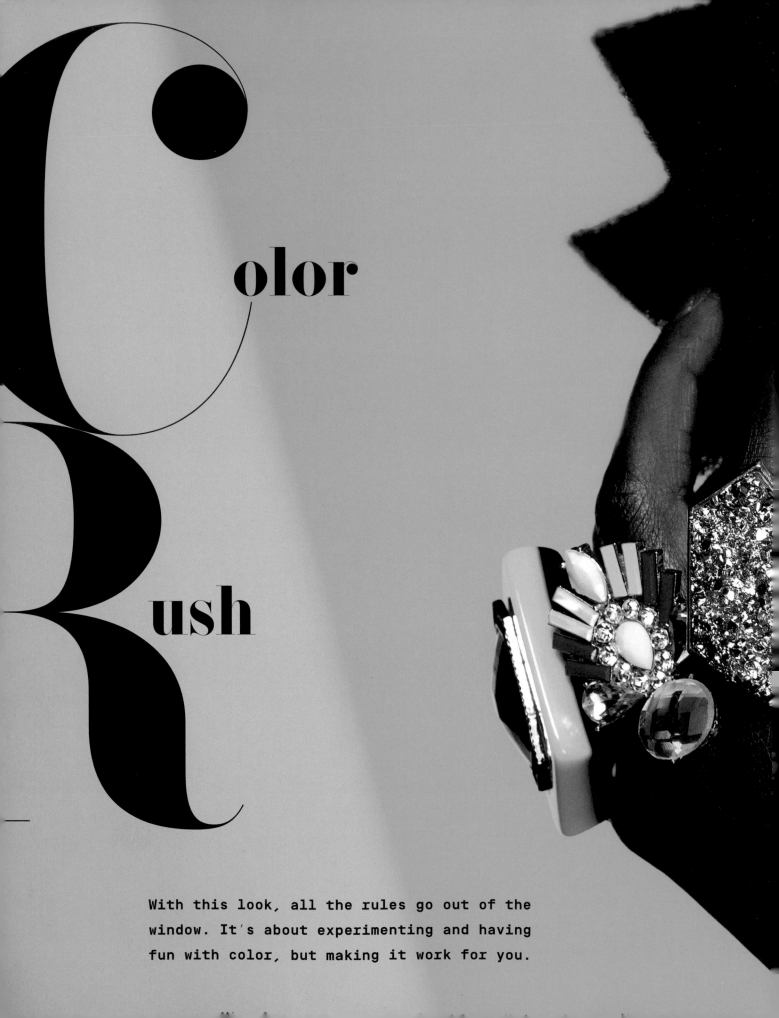

Color Rush

With this look, all the rules go out of the window. It's about experimenting and having fun with color, but making it work for you.

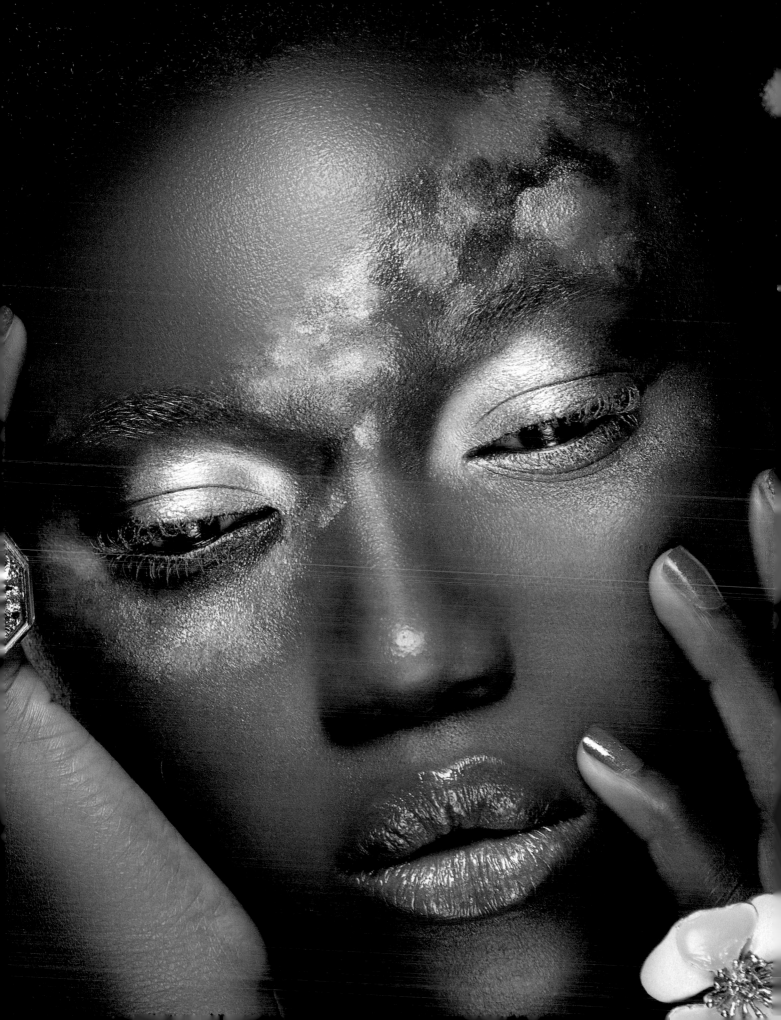

Color Rush Transformation

Working with extreme color is where you can let your creative juices flow and give the artist in you free rein. There are so many eye-popping hues in different textures, tones, and finishes—including high-shine pigment, glitter, and metallic—that you can achieve endless results. Whether you decide to take it to the max or make color work for you in a more restrained way, this is a fun, high-octane look that is going to get you noticed. It's all about expressing yourself and bringing your personality into your make-up, whether that be with sugar-sweet pastels, mouthwatering brights or electric neons.

Strong, vibrant colors will always look effortlessly good on black and olive skin tones. On our model [previous spread], I wanted to take high-fashion color to the edge. Her face has become a canvas that is transformed into an abstract work of art with a bold combination of hues and textures, and while it's not the most wearable look, the effect is dramatic and striking and the message is that make-up is fun and playful. The transformation on Maica was an exercise to see how far I could push the use of color but still create a wearable and beautiful finish that didn't overwhelm her face.

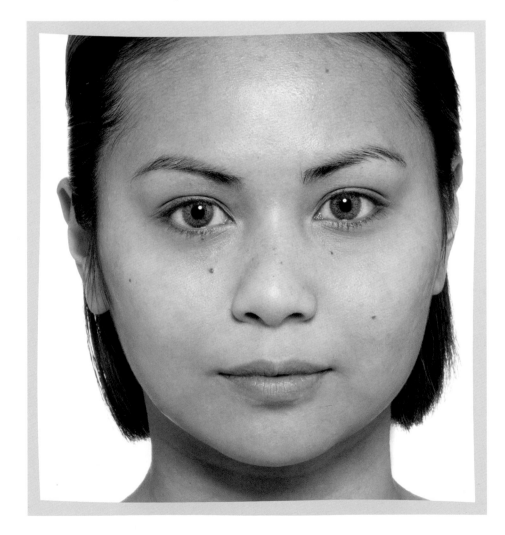

Maica, a dancer in her twenties, has always liked the idea of experimenting with bold colors but tends to stick to classic tones. With her fun, extrovert personality and love of make-up, I knew I could push the boat out with her for this look.

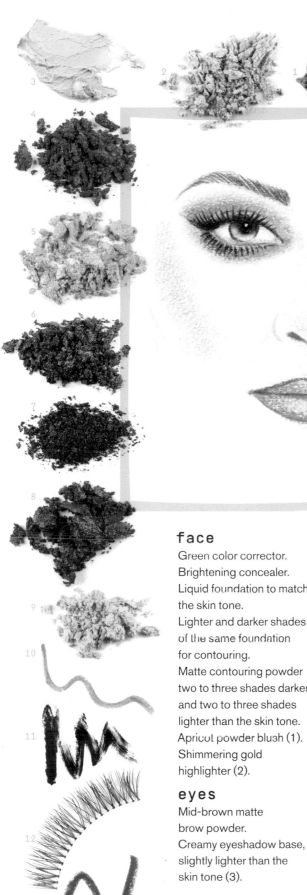

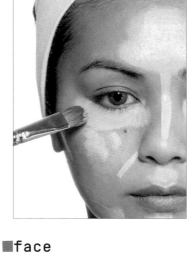

face

Green color corrector.
Brightening concealer.
Liquid foundation to match the skin tone.
Lighter and darker shades of the same foundation for contouring.
Matte contouring powder two to three shades darker and two to three shades lighter than the skin tone.
Apricot powder blush (1).
Shimmering gold highlighter (2).

eyes

Mid-brown matte brow powder.
Creamy eyeshadow base, slightly lighter than the skin tone (3).

Highly pigmented powder eyeshadows in electric-blue (4), bright lime-green (5), hot-pink (6), red (7), orange (8), and canary-yellow (9).
Turquoise pencil eyeliner (10).
Black gel eyeliner (11).
Black mascara.
Strip of feathery false lashes (12).

lips

Creamy crayon lipstick/pencil in a deep, reddish orange (13).
Shimmering gold highlighter (2).

■face

1 After cleansing, toning, and moisturizing, and shaping Maica's brows, I addressed her breakouts by applying green color corrector directly onto her blemishes to counteract the redness. Then I applied a brightening concealer under the eyes and on areas that I wanted to bring forward—the center of the forehead, nose, and chin, above the upper lip, in the nose-to-mouth lines, and under the corners of the mouth.

2 Maica has quite a round face, so after applying a liquid foundation that matched her skin tone, I contoured her face to add structure, using lighter and darker shades of the same foundation (see pages 56–61). I combined and blended them well before using powder to set them.

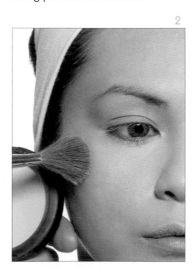

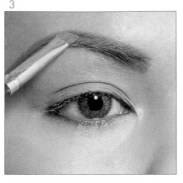

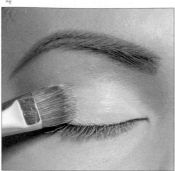

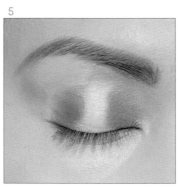

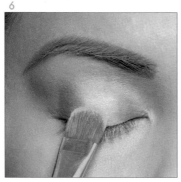

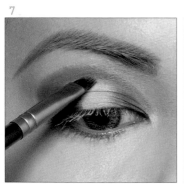

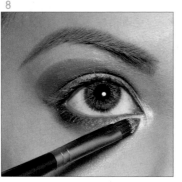

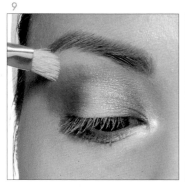

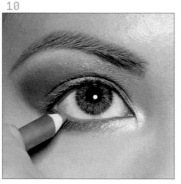

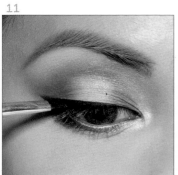

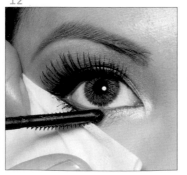

■eyes

3 Her brows were a great shape already, so I just filled them in a little for extra definition with a mid-brown brow powder applied with an angled brush.

4 I applied a creamy eyeshadow base, slightly lighter than her skin tone, all over the lids. This provides a neutral base that makes whatever color you put on top of it stick and look more vibrant.

5 First, I applied an electric-blue powder eyeshadow onto the inner and outer corners of the eyelids, leaving the middle part of the lid clear.

6 Then, using a clean brush, I added a bright lime-green powder eyeshadow in the central section of the eyelids. This vertical section of lighter color makes the eyes look deeper and taller; it draws attention to the mid-section of the eye and makes the eye appear bigger and rounder.

7 Using a small angled brush for precision, I took the electric-blue eyeshadow from the outer corner to the inner corner, slightly higher than the natural crease, to create more space on the eyelid.

8 Using a clean pencil brush for each color, I then created a rainbow of bright colors under the eye, starting with hot-pink on the outer corner, merging through red, to orange, and, finally, to canary-yellow in the inner corner and tear duct.

9 With a soft brush, I added a wash of yellow eyeshadow under the brow bone and blended it into the socket line. If you wish, layer high-shine pigment in the same colors on top.

10 To brighten the eyes and make the whites look whiter, I applied turquoise pencil eyeliner to the waterline.

11 Then I defined the top lash line with black gel liner and drew it out toward the outer corner to lift the eye.

12 I curled the lashes to open up the eyes and applied a little black mascara before adding a strip of feathery false lashes. I added another coat of mascara to the roots of the top lashes to seal the false lashes to them and then applied a coat to the bottom lashes, holding a tissue under the eye to protect the skin from smudges.

> **Tip**
>
> This is a bespoke look that you can tailor to your preference with as many color combinations as you want. Stick to two or three for a subtler look or embrace the rainbow and go for the full color rush.

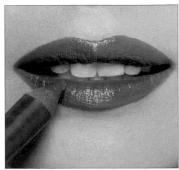

13

■lips

13 I thought bright orange lips would work perfectly with her skin tone for this bold look, so I used a creamy crayon lipstick in a deep, reddish orange and then applied a splash of gold highlighter to the center of the lower lip to add another dimension and bring the look together.

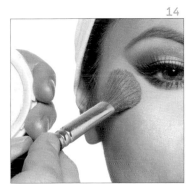

14

■finish

14 To give her face greater definition, I added a little more of the darker shade of contouring powder beneath her cheekbones to push them out slightly further. Then I added warmth to her skin with an apricot powder blush. I also applied gold highlighter on the top of her cheekbones, the beginning of her eyes, above her lip line, and on her neck, décolletage, and shoulders, to bring everything together and give her skin a golden sheen.

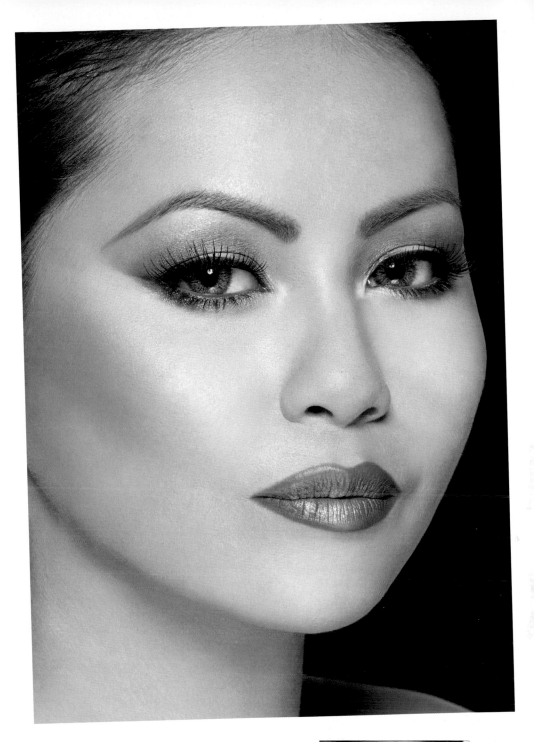

"I don't usually wear a lot of color in everyday life but, as a dancer, I have to when I'm on stage, and I'll definitely use the layering/blending technique that Gary taught me in order to intensify the colors so they stand out more. I'm also very happy that he introduced me to the perfect foundation."

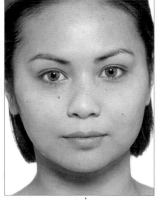

Showgirl

Think glitter and shimmer,
jewel colors and texture—
this is the ultimate party

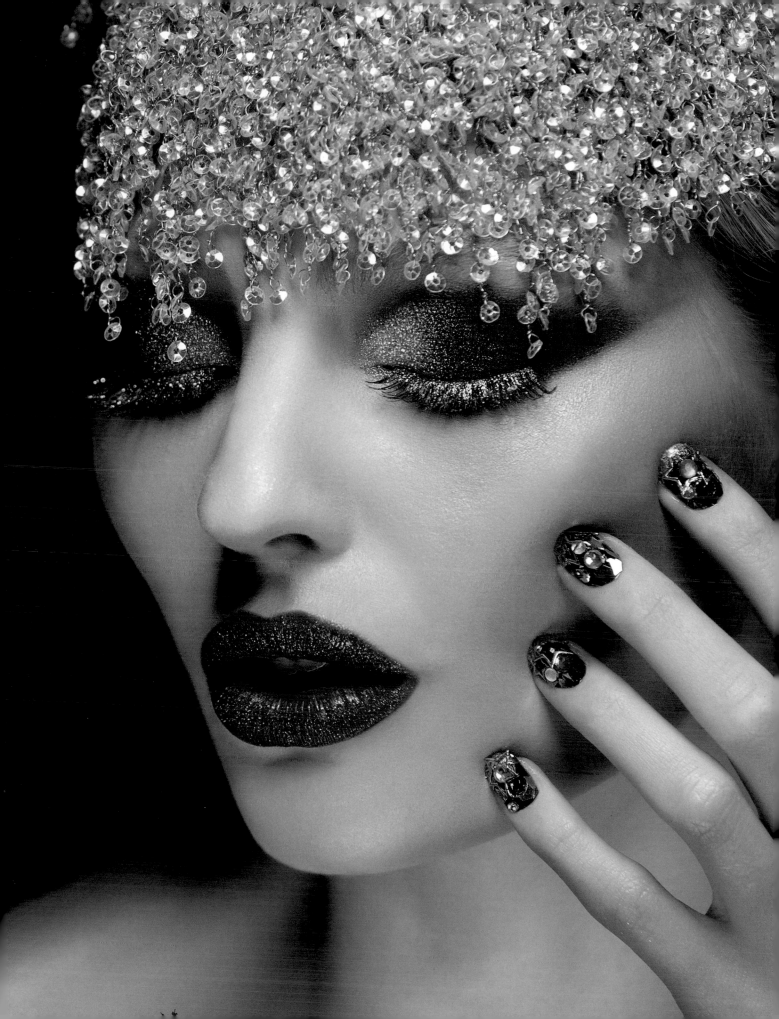

Showgirl Transformation

Everyone needs a touch of sparkle in their life and this high-impact, theatrical look, combining bold colors and shimmery textures, can be a real showstopper. On our model [previous spread], I wanted to demonstrate the ultimate Showgirl look, with a statement eye full of strong colors and high-shine textures topped off with fluttery glitter lashes, and paired with glitter-kissed red lips and rhinestone-embellished nail art. Elle, whom I transformed into a sparkly princess, is only 21, so I could afford to apply a lot of glitter and vibrant color. Her "English rose" complexion could carry off the bright palette and I offset the cool tones with light-reflecting gold pigment and glitter, together with the pretty pinks on her cheeks and lips, which keep the look fresh and youthful. Glitter combined with strong color can be breathtaking, but if it's too much for you, adapt the look with neutral tones [bone, taupe, and brown with black mascara], then add a splash of glitter. If you don't want to use glitter, which is quite grainy, high-impact color pigment gives a similar effect. It sticks to the lid easily and can be used with cream or powder eyeshadow without needing another medium to make it stick.

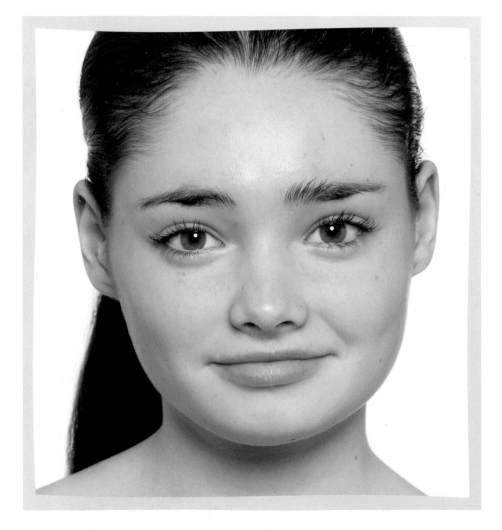

Elle is a pretty girl of 21, whom I knew would make the perfect Showgirl. Not only do the shimmery textures and cool tones suit her young, fair skin, but her bubbly character has as much sparkle as the make-up.

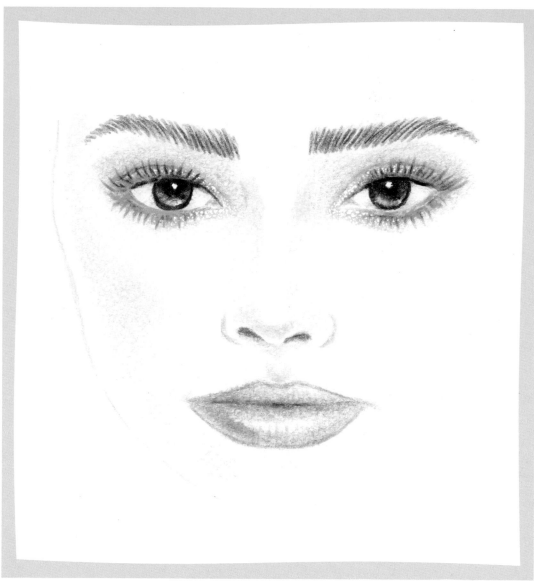

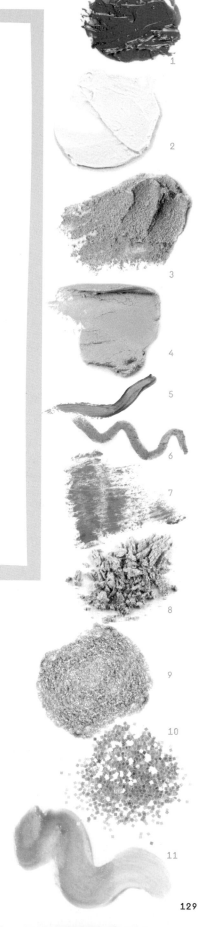

face

Lightweight illuminating primer.
Lightweight liquid foundation.
Pink cream blush (1).

eyes

Light brown matte brow powder.
Cream eyeshadow in a cool
ivory tone (2).
Turquoise cream
eyeshadow (3).
Lime-green cream
eyeshadow (4).
Electric-blue liquid eyeliner (5).
Turquoise pencil eyeliner (6).
Bright blue mascara (7).
High-shine gold pigment (8).
Gold glitter (9).
Glitter gel eyeliner in a light
greenish gold and glitter
particles to match (10).

lips

Creamy, soft pink
lipstick (11).
Clear lip gloss.

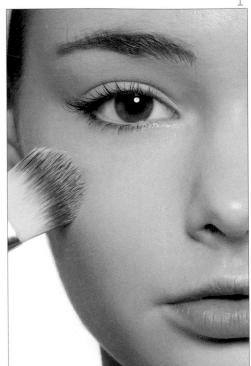

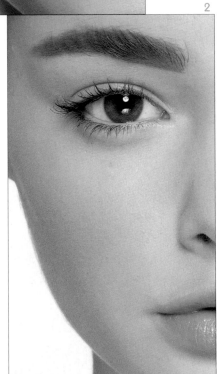

■face

1 After prepping as usual (see pages 28–9), I used an illuminating primer, paying particular attention to her eyelids—priming the eyes is especially important when they are going to have lots of texture on them, as it gives a good base that ensures the eye make-up will last as long as possible. Then I used a lightweight liquid foundation, as I wanted to keep her young skin looking dewy and fresh.

2 To give her cheeks a natural flush, I applied a wash of pink cream blush.

Tip When you have great, youthful skin, make the most of it and keep your make-up lightweight to let the natural glow come through.

■eyes

3 I love the fullness of Elle's eyebrows and wanted to keep them looking very natural. I tweezed them lightly to remove any stray hairs, then brushed them up and filled them in where necessary with a light brown brow powder and an angled brush. Then I applied a cream eyeshadow in a cool ivory tone all over the lid with a medium-sized flat brush.

4 Using the same type of brush, I added a turquoise cream eyeshadow to the outer corner of the eyes.

5 Changing to a small round pencil brush, I took the same turquoise eyeshadow into the crease of the eye and just above it, blending it into the ivory base on the lid.

6 I then swept the turquoise under the eye from the outer edge to the inner corner.

7 With another pencil brush, I added a touch of lime-green cream eyeshadow under the lower lash line at the inner corner of the eye, and blended it into the turquoise.

8 I applied electric-blue liquid eyeliner along the upper lash line, just on the roots of the lashes, to frame the eyes and add depth.

9 Next, I applied a turquoise pencil eyeliner to the lower waterline.

10 I coated the top and bottom lashes with bright blue mascara, working the wand from the roots to the tips to color the lashes blue.

11 To add the showgirl shimmer, I first applied a high-shine gold pigment onto the first part of the eyelid, taking it from the inner corner and fading it toward the middle section of the lid. Pigment travels, so add a very little at a time and build it up gradually so that it doesn't overpower the eye. Then, using a flat brush, I pressed a little gold glitter on top of this to give a champagne-colored sparkly texture.

12 To finish the eyes, I used a glitter gel liner and loose glitter particles in a light greenish gold underneath the lower lash line, starting at the inner corner and taking it to the middle, so the focus is drawn to the beginning of the eyes.

13 Finally, I added a touch of the same gel liner and glitter to the mid-section of the eyelid to accentuate that area even more.

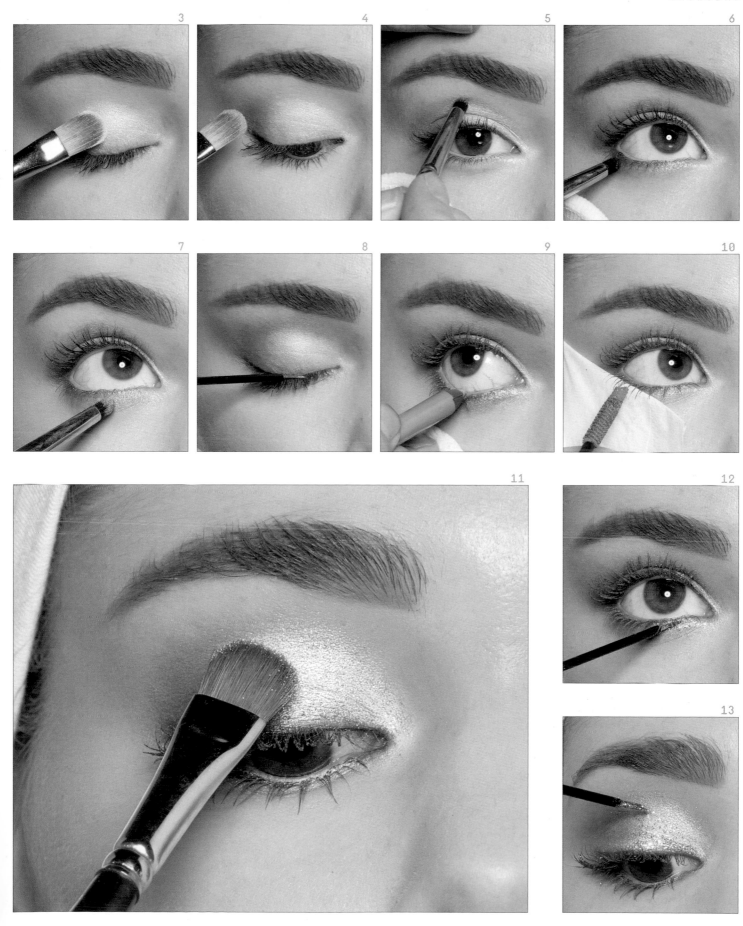

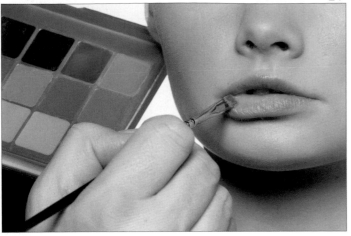

14

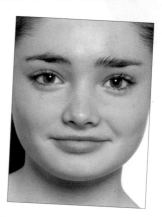

"I loved this look. It had a young, fresh and glamorous feel—perfect for a fabulous party night out. Gary gave me a flawless porcelain complexion and natural glossy lips, which allowed the most striking sparkly eye make-up I've ever worn to stand out. I felt like Anna from Frozen—I felt wonderful."

■lips

14 All the drama is on the eyes and I didn't want to detract from this, so I finished the lips with a creamy lipstick in a soft pink and a hint of gloss on the bottom lip.

glitter application

» Glitter can be messy, so use a glue, gel, or mixing medium to help fix it in place.

» Applying a creamy eyeshadow as a base ensures the glitter will stick to the lid when it's applied with a flat eyeshadow brush or your fingertips.

» If glitter drops on your face, use low-tack masking tape to lift it off the skin without smudging your foundation.

» If you're creating a heavy-duty glitter look, do your eyes before your foundation in case of fallout [see also page 115].

» To remove glitter, use a water- or oil-based cleanser. Glitter has a coarse texture, so use gentle strokes and be careful not to get it in your eye.

thoughts on glitter looks

» Add a touch of glitter to any party, prom, festival, or festive make-up, as it may be the finishing touch that really sets your look apart. Glitter lashes and rhinestones will take the look to the next level.

» Glitter can be worn by women of all ages, depending on your eye shape, how much you apply, and where you apply it. A full-on glitter eye works better on fuller lids, as high-shine texture draws attention to hooded lids and lines. Older eyes can be given a hint of sparkle with a sweep of glitter liner along the upper lash line.

» Keep to light shades of glitter—anything too dark can make the eyes look hard and the skin look dull.

» Going too mad with glitter can overwhelm the eyes. So to keep it wearable and flattering, focus on the mid-section or the first half of the eyelid to create drama with a contrast of light and dark, or use a glitter liner along the lash line.

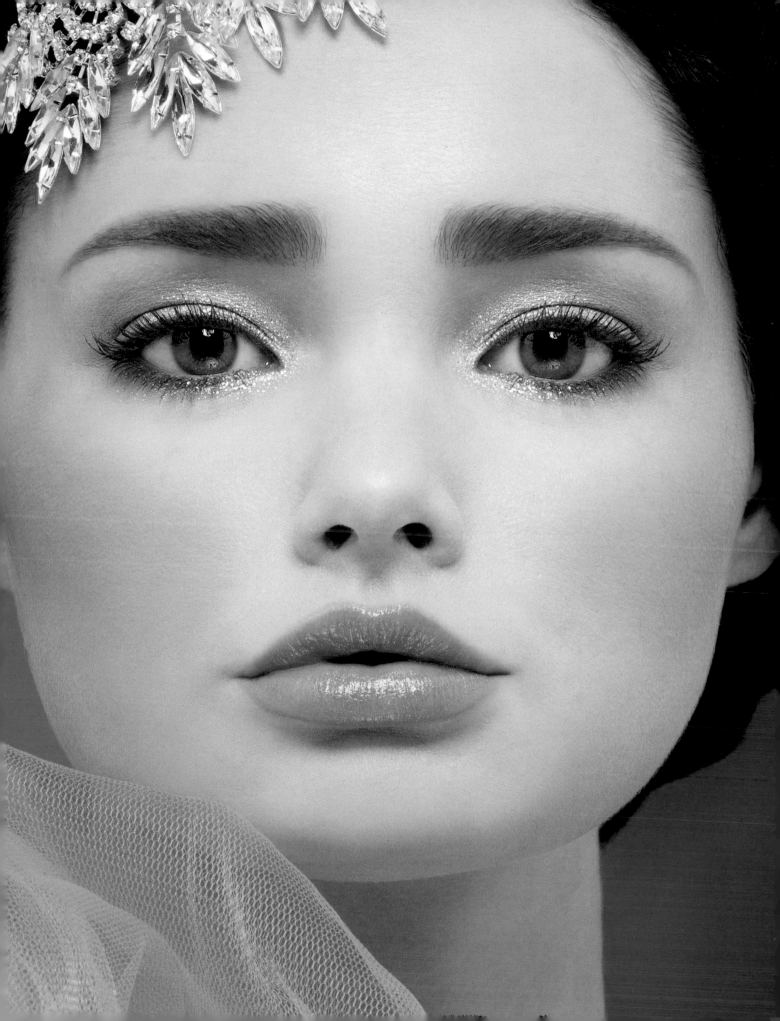

Mascara

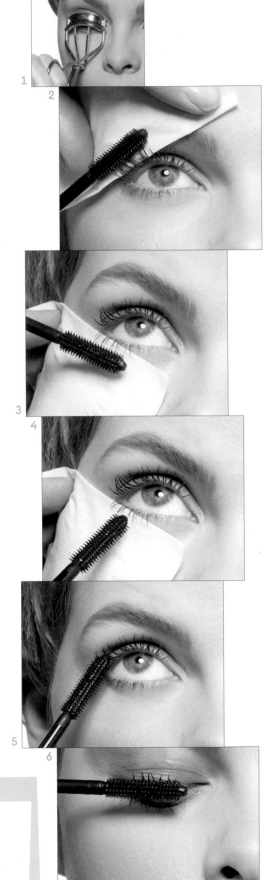

Flirty, fluttery eyelashes frame the eyes and finish off any look, but most people weren't born with naturally fabulous lashes. Curling the lashes opens up the eyes and changes their shape, while mascara makes the lashes look fuller, longer, and defined.

1 Curling the lashes not only opens up the eyes but also creates a great shape before applying mascara. I usually do this in three stages. Take your eyelash curlers and, starting right at the roots, clamp the lashes firmly but gently for 7–10 squeezes, then release. Move the curlers to the mid-section of the lashes and repeat. Finally, go right to the tips of the lashes and give them 7–10 squeezes. This produces a gentle curve and ensures all the lashes are going in the right direction. If your lashes don't curl easily, heat the curlers for a few seconds with your hairdryer—test them on the back of your hand to make sure the metal isn't too hot.

2 Place the mascara wand horizontally beneath the upper lashes, as close to the roots as possible, and slowly pull it up to the mid-length, then lighten the pressure and wiggle it from side to side as you pull it through the ends of the lashes. Holding a tissue on the other side of the lashes ensures you don't catch the skin and also means you can see each lash individually so you know exactly how much mascara you've applied.

3 Holding a tissue under the eye to prevent smudges, apply mascara to the bottom lashes. (The eye area is very delicate so don't rub the skin.)

4 Turn the wand vertically to separate the lashes, remove any clumps, and ensure all the lashes are coated with mascara.

5 Do the same with the upper lashes and apply more mascara to the roots to add depth, using the tip of the wand for precision.

6 Turn the wand horizontally again and wiggle it from side to side, working the mascara through the upper lashes, coating the sides and roots for more fullness, and layering it to create the desired finish.

how to create more definition

» For extra definition, paint dark gel liner along the lash line and the base of the lashes before applying mascara.

» Tightlining—where you dot dark brown or black eyeliner pencil between the roots of the lashes, top and bottom— adds depth and makes sparse lashes look fuller and thicker.

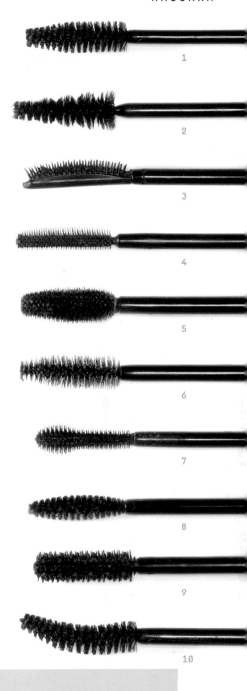

magic wands

Whether spiral, pine-tree shaped, curved, conical, or spherical, the size and shape of a mascara wand really do matter, as wands are specially designed to achieve different results, such as thickening, volumizing, lengthening, curling, or fanning out the lashes. Some are better than others at reaching different parts of the eye, such as the roots of the lashes, the bottom lashes, shorter lashes, or the corners. The bristles may be nylon, plastic, rubber, silicone, or hair, and they may be short or long, densely packed or spaced apart.

1 Mid-size, natural-bristle, spiral wand This is good for lengthening, separating, and defining the lashes.

2 Precision spiral wand The thinner end allows for precision; this wand coats the lashes thoroughly.

3 Rubber shorty wand This defines, lengthens, and combs the lashes to prevent clogging while coating every lash for a natural finish. It makes the lashes fan out and is good for reaching the inner corners.

4 Micro wand This small, slim brush is good for short lashes, bottom lashes, and picking out detail. It gives natural definition and is good for working vertically.

5 Oversized wand This large, fat wand carries a lot of product so it really coats the lashes and creates maximum volume and impact.

6 Natural-bristle wand The fine hairs coat the lashes with mascara really well, giving good, natural-looking coverage.

7 Bald-tip wand This allows great precision and is good for creating detail and defining short and corner lashes.

8 Conical wand This is designed to get to the base of the lashes and define short lashes.

9 Flat comb wand This separates lashes but gives great volume, helping to make the eyes look bigger.

10 Curved wand This curls, lifts, and fans out the lashes.

Tips

» To avoid clumping, wipe the wand with a tissue to get rid of excess mascara before applying it.

» To give the lashes more density and direction, change the angle when applying mascara and use different-shaped wands for different effects.

» Mascara expands as it dries, so let it dry and then comb through with a metal lash comb in between coats.

» Try not to pump the wand in and out of the tube, as this will make the mascara dry out.

» Replace mascara every three months, as a build-up of bacteria can cause eye infections.

» Have fun with mascara—try different colors or pull out all the stops with a glitter finish.

False lashes

Fake lashes take your make-up to a whole new level and are essential for creating the ultimate glamorous eyes. Soft and natural or full and heavy, they are the perfect way to enhance your eyes and customize your look. Whether you choose full strip lashes, corner lashes, clusters, or individual lashes, they will accentuate, elongate, and open up the eyes.

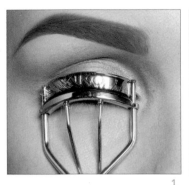
1

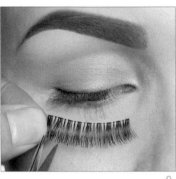
2

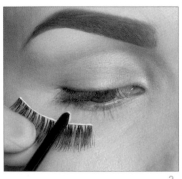
3

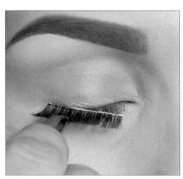
4

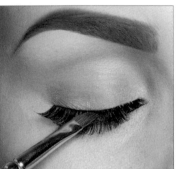
5

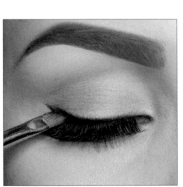
6

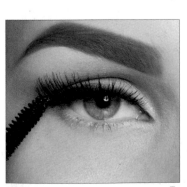
7

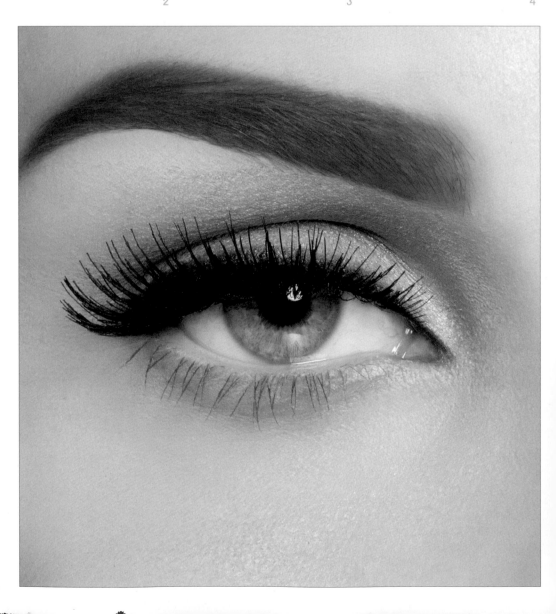

strip lashes

When people think of false lashes, they usually think of strip lashes, such as this full, fluttery set (opposite). Choose lashes made of real (not synthetic) hair, with an invisible strip—the more delicate the strip is, the more pliable and natural the lashes will be.

1 Curl your lashes.

2 Holding the false lashes with tweezers or your fingers, place them over the lash line to check whether the strip is the right size. If you need to, trim it from the outer edge, then place it back on the eye and check that it fits.

3 Most lashes come with glue, so apply it generously to the back of the strip—I use the end of a thin brush to spread it evenly. Make sure you put plenty of glue on both ends—if the strip is going to lift, it will do so at the ends first.

4 The most important thing is to let the glue get tacky before you stick the strip in place, otherwise it will slide around. Wait 8–10 seconds and then apply it to your lash line with tweezers.

5 Push it in place with a small angled brush or tweezers, as close to the roots of your natural lashes as you can. Don't use a Q-tip, as the fibers will shed and get stuck in the glue.

6 When the glue is dry and the lashes are secure, add eyeliner along the top of the lash line to "seal" the join and create depth.

7 Apply mascara from the roots upward, so the natural lashes blend with the false ones.

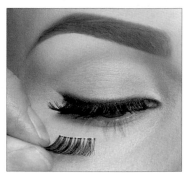

8

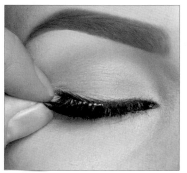

9

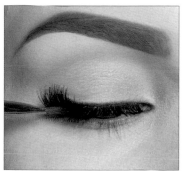

10

corner lashes

Enhancing the outer part of the eye, corner lashes (this page) are great for feline looks or close-set eyes, as they lift, elongate, and pull the eyes apart. They create a more natural, less intense look than a full lash and are the perfect complement to a fifties flick. You can also use them to create extreme drama by layering them over strip lashes to give more of a kick at the end, as I have here.

8 If you are using corner lashes on their own, curl your natural lashes and apply a coat of mascara first. Decide where you are going to position the corner lashes—don't place them right at the corner, as this will give the effect of a down-turned eye rather than creating "lift."

9 Apply glue to the back of the strip and wait 8–10 seconds for it to become tacky. Using your fingers or tweezers, place the false lashes on the last three-quarters of the lid, a fraction in from the end of your lash line.

10 Press the lashes firmly in place with a small angled brush or tweezers. When the glue is dry, push the lashes up from underneath before adding eyeliner, if you wish.

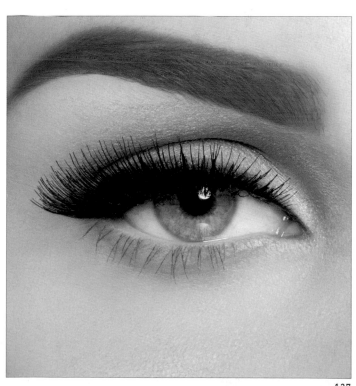

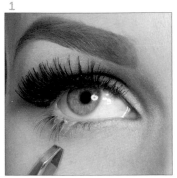

1

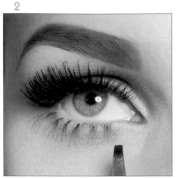

2

bottom lashes

For a really wide-eyed look, you can buy ready-made bottom lashes on transparent strips, but I prefer to use individual lashes (this page, left), as you can decide where to place them to change the shape of your eye. Black lashes are too heavy underneath the eyes, so go for dark brown and choose short, medium, or long lashes, depending on your eye shape and the look you are trying to create—your eye will dictate what it can take. They are not easy to apply, so practice before the big night.

1 Holding the lashes with tweezers or your fingers, apply glue to the root.

2 If you're creating an elongated eye, start at the outer corner and work in (as I did here). For a rounder eye, start in the middle with the longest lashes and work outward. There's no need to add mascara.

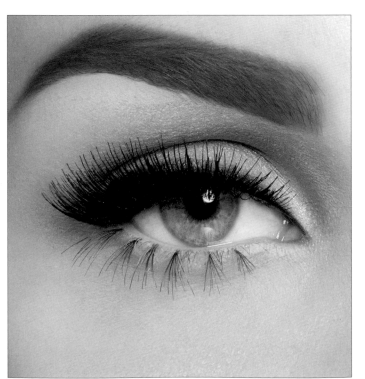

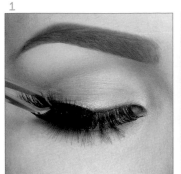

1

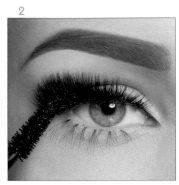

2

ultimate lashes

Layer up your false lashes to create the ultimate 3-D lashes (this page, right). Start with a medium-length, fluttery strip, then cut another strip in half and add it to the second half of the eye. Finally, add some clusters or a corner lash to the outer edge of the eye for extra va-va-voom. This is a better way to create a really extreme look than applying one full-on set, as you can customize them to your eye shape and stop when you wish. This look may not work for everyone—if you've got fine features or light brows, choose finer lashes in brown, rather than black, for a softer look. It can be too much to add bottom lashes as well, but I have here to show the "X-Factor" of lash looks.

1 Add each strip, half-strip, and cluster as before.

2 Wait for the glue to dry and push the lashes up before adding the next set. After the last lash is firmly in place, apply mascara to the roots to blend the layers together.

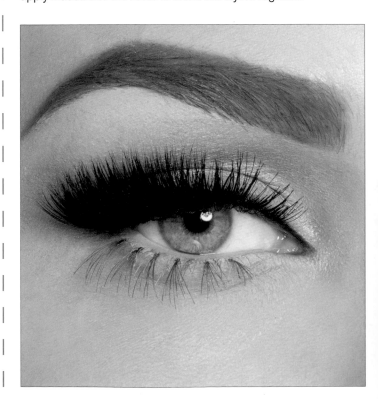

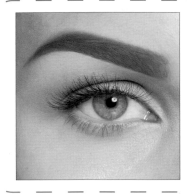

individual lashes and clusters

Single lashes or flares of lashes subtly enhance your natural lashes for a softer, minimal look (left). They come in short, medium, and long, and you can add as many or as few as you wish, tailoring them to the effect you want to achieve. Use them to fill in gaps or to add thickness and fullness to your natural lashes, or to give a little more definition to a strip lash. You can use them on the bottom lash line as well as the top. Apply a dot of glue to the end and use tweezers to position them as you wish.

removing lashes

Starting at the outer corner of the eye, lift the edge of the strip from your lash line and carefully peel it off. If the glue is stubborn, use a little make-up remover or almond oil to soften it. Always take false lashes off before removing the rest of your eye make-up and never sleep in them.

Tips

» You can customize a lash strip by cutting it into several sections. Keep them in the correct order, so the longest lashes are at the outer corner or in the center, depending on the shape of lashes you've chosen, and place them on your lash line at very slightly different angles, with a little space between each section. This will give a lighter, more natural look than a full strip lash and you can customize the eye by adding more to the mid-section or outer corner.

» Always curl your own lashes before you apply false ones.

» Apply a dark eyeliner pencil or dark matte eyeshadow along your upper lash line at the base of the lashes before applying false lashes, to create depth and density. This also hides any gaps if you don't get the lashes in exactly the right place.

» To create maximum thickness and fullness, apply mascara before you put the false lashes on; once they are in place, apply a little more just to the roots, to blend your natural lashes with the false ones.

» Eyelash glue often contains Latex, so check the box and do a skin test to make sure you don't have any adverse reactions.

» Position the false lashes a fraction in from the end of your lash line; if the false lashes overhang the eye, they will drag it down and make it look straight and deep-set.

» When you've attached the false lashes, bend them up with the tip of your finger before you open your eye.

» If you have unruly lashes, apply mascara after you've put the false lashes on; you can then "stick" your natural lashes onto the false ones with the tip of your mascara wand so they'll all lie in the right direction and look more natural.

» Look after your false lashes, as you should be able to get a few wears out of them. Peel off the glue, using eye make-up remover if necessary, and store them in their original packaging.

» To create a rounder eye, use false lashes that are longer in the middle.

» To create a feline eye, use false lashes that are longer at the outer edge to elongate the eye.

» If you have small eyes, choose lightweight false lashes, as anything too heavy will overwhelm and close the eyes.

Precious metal

High-impact metallics are never out of fashion and there are many ways to wear them, whether as a soft wash for the daytime or a shimmering statement for the evening.

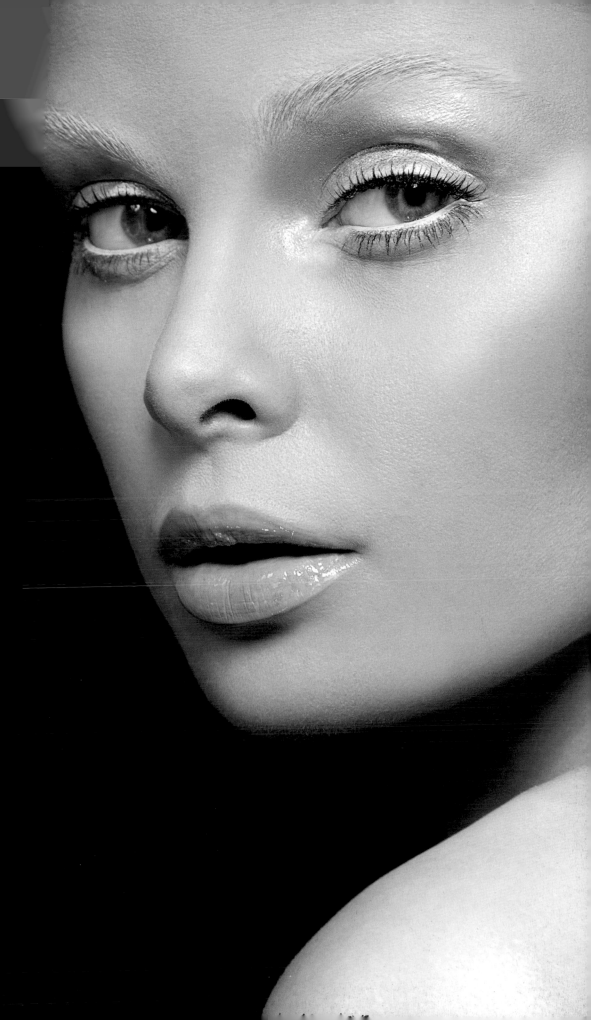

Precious Metal Transformation

I love metallics, whether cool silver and pewter or warm gold and bronze, as they reflect light and create drama and depth. They are great to use as highlighters and are the perfect way to add intensity to a look. Metallic eyeshadows come in the form of cream, powder, and pigment; there are also metallic eyeliners, which can be used alone or in combination with other metallic products, and foils, which can be applied over eyeshadow on the beginning or mid-section of the eye for a dramatic 3-D effect. Picking the right tone is key to achieving a great statement look that isn't too harsh or "alien." The convention is that silvery shades look better on cool, fair skin tones and gold and bronze look better on warm, olive skin tones. To complement our model's cool, porcelain skin [previous spread], I applied a simple silver metallic wash on the lid using cream eyeshadow. With Hari, who has a lovely medium skin, I challenged the "rule" by showing that adding a warm tone to the socket line and blending it well into the silver base softens the look and tones down the harshness of the cool silver. The result was a dramatic, smoky, cat's eye that really made the most of her eyes. Never be afraid to try anything and experiment to see how you can make a look, color, or texture work for you.

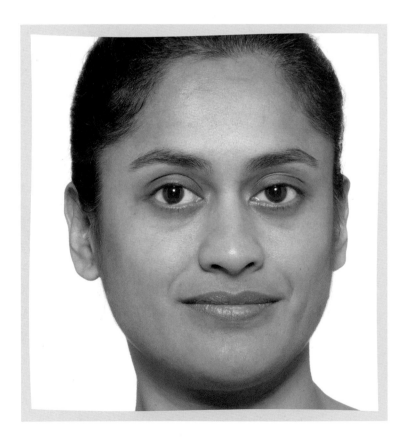

Hari is in her thirties and I wanted to prove that metallics can suit anyone, no matter what the "rules" of make-up suggest, so I created a metallic cat's eye to elongate and widen her eyes, and warmed up the cool silver with a base layer of soft brown.

face
High-definition hydrating primer.
Lightweight liquid foundation to match the skin tone.
Darker and lighter cream foundation for contouring.
Translucent powder.
Powder blush in a soft pink (1).
Champagne highlighter (2).

eyes
Light brown matte brow powder.
Warm brown matte powder eyeshadow (3).
Silver cream eyeshadow (4).
Vanilla powder eyeshadow (5).
Silver pigment eyeshadow (6).
Dark silver-gray matte powder eyeshadow (7).
Black gel eyeliner (8).
Black matte powder eyeshadow (9).
Black mascara.
Clusters of feathery false lashes (10).
Black pencil eyeliner (11).

lips
Nude lip liner (12).
Pink-toned, nude, creamy lipstick (13).
Clear lip gloss.

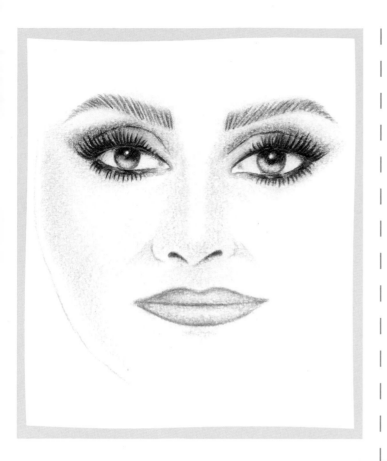

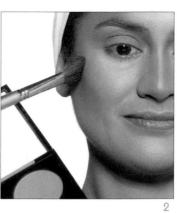

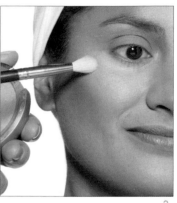

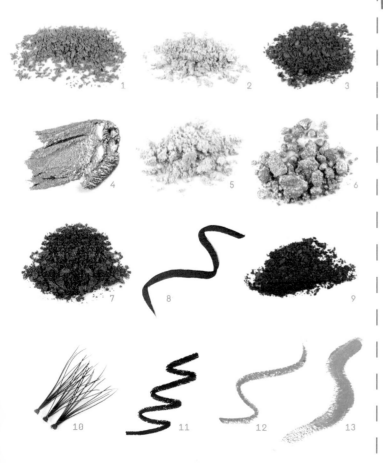

■face

1 After prepping and priming (see pages 28–9), paying special attention to the eyes to make the eyeshadows last longer, I applied a light liquid foundation to match her skin tone. A metallic eye is a strong look and works well with light, daytime make-up on the face, so contouring is optional. I wanted to give Hari's face more dimension and structure, so I applied a darker cream foundation to slim down her nose, carve out her cheekbones, make her forehead smaller, and sculpt her jaw (see pages 56–61).

2 I applied a lighter cream foundation to the areas I wanted to highlight, especially under the eyes, along the brow bones and the center of the nose, and on the forehead, chin, and upper lip. I blended it well and set it with powder.

3 I then brought warmth to the cheeks with powder blush in a soft pink.

4 A matte face looks out of place with high-shine eyes—you want the skin to look illuminated and slightly shimmery, but with warm tones to counteract the coolness of the metallics. I added a touch of highlighter in a champagne tone above the cheekbones and other areas I wanted to bring forward, such as the beginning of the eye, the upper lip, and the chin.

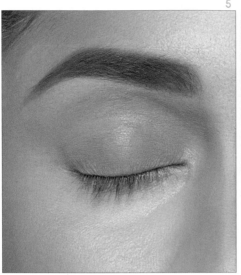

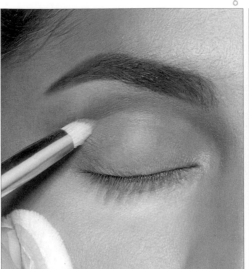

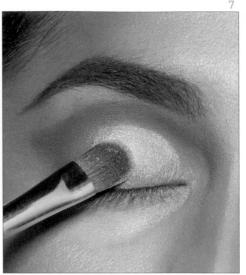

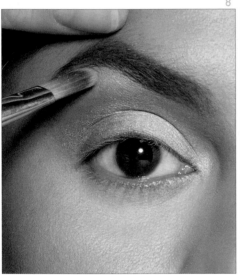

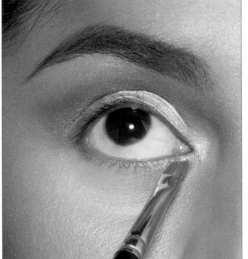

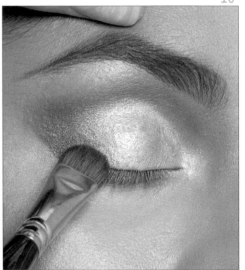

■ eyes

5 Hari's brows were a great shape, so I just neatened them with a light brown matte brow powder. I kept them slightly lighter than her hair color so as not to draw attention away from the eyes themselves or overpower her face—there's nothing worse than heavy, black eyebrows that make you look like Groucho Marx.

6 Adding warm tones to the eyes as a base for this look ensures the cool metallic won't seem too harsh when it hits the skin. Using a small pencil brush, I cut out a crease with warm brown matte eyeshadow along Hari's

socket line—as her eyes are naturally big and round, I didn't need to cheat by taking the crease line any higher.

7 I applied a silver cream eyeshadow onto the main part of the eyelid.

8 To add more warmth, I brushed a vanilla powder eyeshadow just beneath her brow bone. When blended together where they meet, the warm tones above the socket and the cool ones below create a lovely finish.

9 I then added the silver cream eyeshadow to the inner corner of the eye and swept it under the waterline with a small angled brush.

10 I layered a high-impact, silver pigment eyeshadow over the cream, pressing it onto the lid with a flat brush to make it stick well. To build the drama, I applied a darker silver-gray matte powder eyeshadow to the outer corners and blended it into the light silver pigment on the lid and the warm brown in the socket line. I also swept it under the lash line at the outer corner of the eye to help pull the eyes apart.

11 Then I applied black gel liner along the upper lash line, using a small angled brush. I made the line thin at the beginning of the eye and thickened

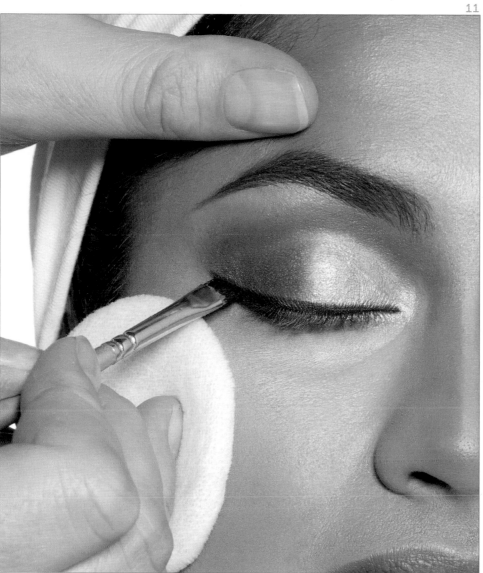

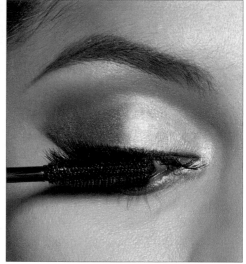

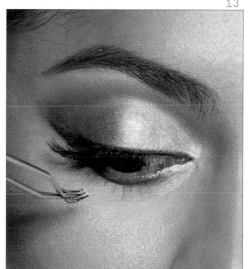

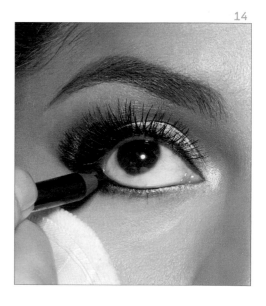

it toward the outer edge, flicking it up at the outer corner toward the end of her brow to create a cat's-eye effect that really pulls the eyes apart. I then went over the liner with black matte powder eyeshadow, which helps to set it and gives a softer line.

12–13 I curled the upper lashes and applied a little black mascara. Then I added clusters of feathery false

lashes from the outer edge of the eye working inward, putting more lashes at the outer edges to draw her eyes apart (see page 139). Then I applied more mascara, but only to the roots of the lashes for added depth, and to the bottom lashes.

14 To finish the eyes, I applied black pencil liner inside and around the waterline, top and bottom.

> **Tip** For a more natural look with false lashes, don't apply mascara to the full length, but just to the roots for added depth and drama.

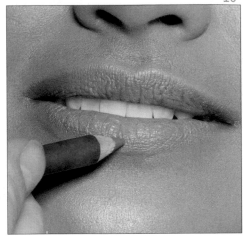

15

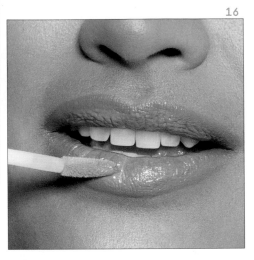

16

■lips

15 I wanted to focus all the drama on her eyes and keep her lips very natural, so I primed them first with a little foundation to cancel out any natural pigment in her lips that would alter the color of the lipstick, and then I lined her lips with a nude lip pencil.

16 I applied a pink-toned, nude, creamy lipstick with a brush and added a hint of gloss to the middle of the bottom lip to catch the light and make the lips look fuller.

Remember:

Applying foundation or concealer
to the lips first ensures the
lipstick will be true to color.

how to master metallic eyeshadow

» For a quick, easy-to-wear metallic look, use a cream-based eyeshadow on the lid and blend it outward until it fades to transparent on the skin.

» If you're wary of cream eyeshadows because of their tendency to crease, try a wash of powder eyeshadow, which gives a soft, understated finish.

» For a more extreme, high-shine look, apply metallic pigment over the wash, but use a cream eyeshadow base to give it something to adhere to for greater staying power.

» When you are applying any sort of metallic finish to the eye, always use an eyeshadow primer on the lid first to create a good base that will help to keep it in place.

» Metallic eyeshadows that can be used dry or wet are a good investment. Use them dry for a subtle powder finish or dip the brush in water for a more intense look. Apply it over the whole lid or just on the upper lash line.

» Metallic cream-to-powder eyeshadow goes on like cream and looks like cream on the eye, but dries to a powdery consistency for a longer-lasting, crease-free, creamy finish.

» Metallics can be used to highlight the mid-section of the lid, the beginning of the eye and around the waterline, and beneath the brow bone.

» Gold tones look fantastic with red lips, whereas silver tones work best with a natural, pinky nude lip.

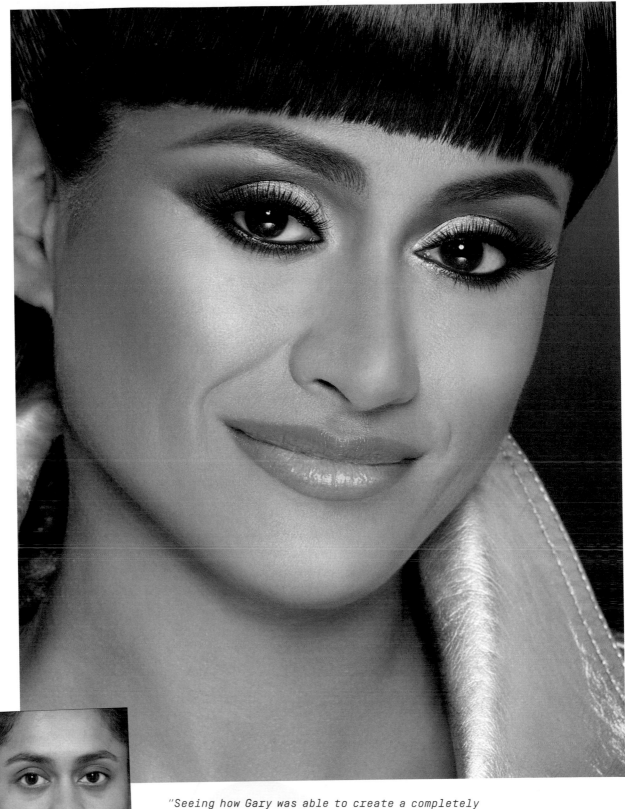

"Seeing how Gary was able to create a completely new look for me was amazing and the contouring was unbelievable, making me look young and fresh again. I had thought metallic eye make-up was a bit young for me, but watching Gary apply it made me realize that this is something I could do for a dramatic, yet elegant evening look."

For defining the eyes, changing their shape, or creating impact, nothing beats eyeliner. Whether it's a soft line of shadow to add depth, an exaggerated flick to elongate the eye, or a sweep of color, metallic, or glitter to make a statement, eyeliner allows you to change the mood of the eyes in an instant. Different colors, textures, and applications can be used on the waterline, lash line, or both to create a range of stunning effects, from subtle, to sexy, to dramatic.

eyeliner

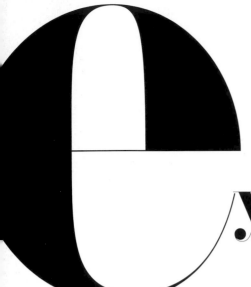

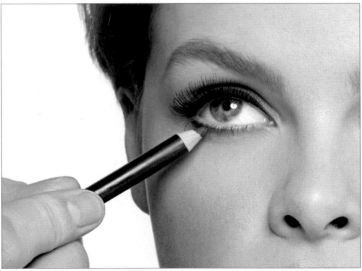

1 2
3 4

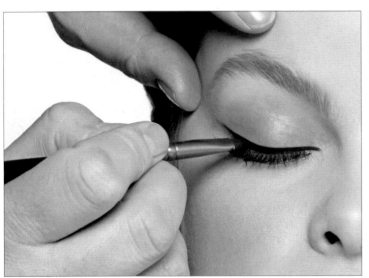

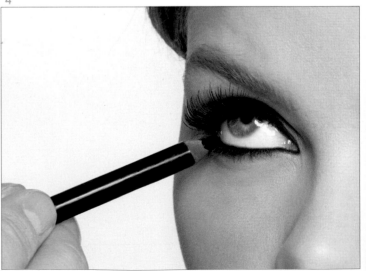

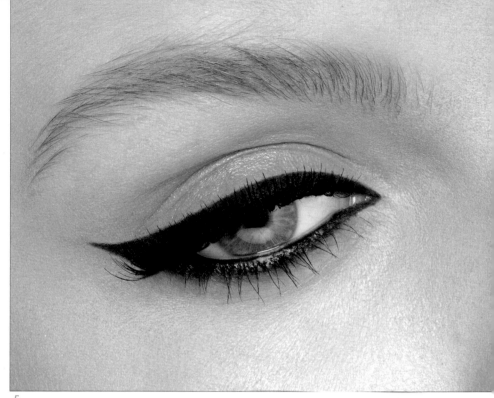

1 A great way to define and elongate the eyes is to apply eyeliner along the upper lash line and create a feline flick. Apply black gel liner with a small angled brush for a precise, clean line. Build up the line from the inner corner of the eye toward the outer corner, keeping it softer at the beginning and deeper at the outer corner. To lift the eye, extend the line beyond the corner of your eye, flicking it upward just before you reach the end of your eye.

2 To add more definition, line the lower lash line with a soft eye pencil, working the color into the roots of the lashes. I always go for a slightly lighter tone for beneath the eyes, such as a mid-brown, as black can look too hard.

3 A nude or off-white creamy pencil applied to the lower waterlines will help to brighten and wake up tired eyes and make the whites of your eyes look whiter—unless they are bloodshot, in which case it can do the opposite. Choose a warm tone that isn't too stark white, as this will look unnatural. You can apply the pencil all the way along the waterline, keeping it softer at the beginning of the eye (as I did here), or only beneath the iris to draw attention to the color of your eye.

4 To dress the eyes up for a maximum-impact evening look, coat the waterline with soft black kohl pencil. This gives a sultry feel and looks great on dark brown, blue, or green eyes as it really makes them pop. You can just line the bottom waterline or go all around the eye to add more intensity.

5 This sexy, wearable feline flick makes the eye look larger and more dynamic. It's created with the key combination of liners (1, 2, and 3), with a subtle apricot eyeshadow and a few coats of mascara to finish it off. You can wear this style of eyeliner with or without eyeshadow and vary it in the degree of application, according to the effect you want to achieve.

5

Tips

» Pull the lid taut as you apply eyeliner to the top of the eye to keep the line clean and crisp.

» To prevent the line from looking severe, soften the edges with a small angled brush or a Q-tip.

» For a soft but intense finish, apply powder eyeshadow on top of pencil or gel liner.

» For really soft definition and depth around the eye, apply powder eyeshadow to the lash lines.

» Choose a soft, creamy eyeliner pencil, as you don't want anything too hard that will drag the skin. Keep it sharp, but slightly blunt the tip on the back of your hand before applying it.

» Only use liquid eyeliner if you want a strong, solid line. It's not the easiest thing to apply, and if you make a mistake, it's hard to correct.

» If you have small eyes, don't apply eyeliner all the way around the eyes, especially on the waterline, as it can make them look even smaller.

» If you have dark eyes or a dark skin tone, lining the top waterlines will make the eyes pop, but this can look hard if you have very fair skin and pale eyes.

» Glitter or metallic liners offer an easy way to dress up the eyes, while colored eyeliners along the lower waterlines or upper lash lines are great for experimenting with color.

Perfect flick

A fabulous feline flick, which frames and elongates the eyes while lifting the outer corners, flatters everyone and is a great way to make a statement. It's a bold, confident look that is about showing you're in control and getting noticed. It's also utterly timeless and can be seen on female icons in every decade, from Audrey Hepburn to Kate Moss.

I recommend cream or gel liner for this look, as pencil liner is either too soft or too hard and tends to create a broken line, while liquid liner is high-maintenance, messy, and difficult to apply. Your key tools are a small angled brush and a steady hand.

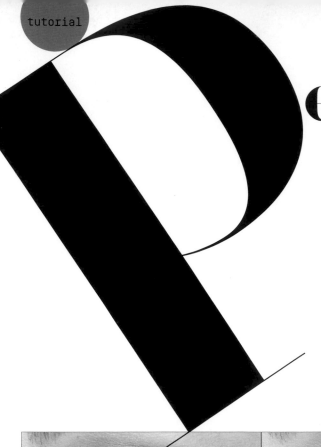

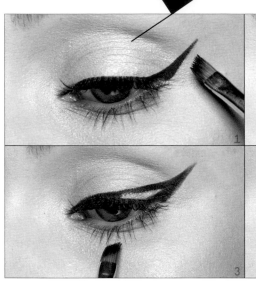

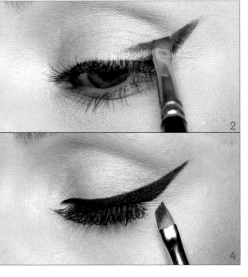

Tips

» Keep Q-tips and eye make-up remover at hand to clean up any mistakes.

» Perfecting the most flattering angle for your eye shape will give you a mini eyelift, but if the flick is too straight, it will drag the eye down and make you look tired.

1 Looking in a mirror, draw a line along the upper lash line and extend it upward and outward from the outer corner of your eye to the point where you want the flick to end. This will depend on what suits your eye shape (see page 94) and how bold you want the flick to be. Try to do this in one sweep, keeping the line as straight as possible and at the desired angle. If you find it easier, put a dot where you want the flick to end and take the line out from the corner of your eye to that point.

2 Still looking in the mirror, tilt your head back and draw another line down from the tip you've just created toward the mid-section of the eye, curving it slightly but keeping the line clean.

3 Take that line along the lash line, all the way to the beginning of the eye, tapering it to make it thinner from the mid-section onward.

4 Check that each line is as sharp as possible and then fill in the triangle space in between, creating a bold, dramatic flick.

Repeat on the other eye, matching the flick as closely as you can.

→ This striking, statement flick looks great with nothing more than a soft, neutral eyeshadow, mascara, and a little highlighter under perfectly groomed brows. But if you wish, you can take it further by lengthening and thickening the flick, or dressing it up with liner under the eyes and false lashes. Finish with a soft blush on the cheeks and either nude or bold lips, depending on how far you want to push it.

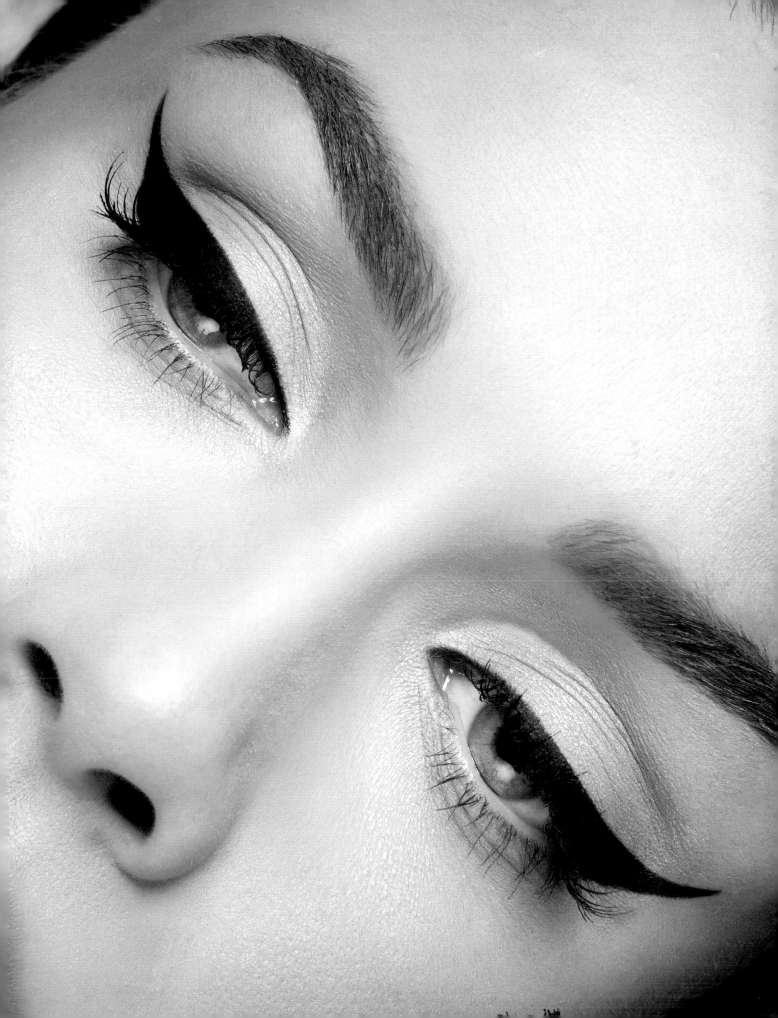

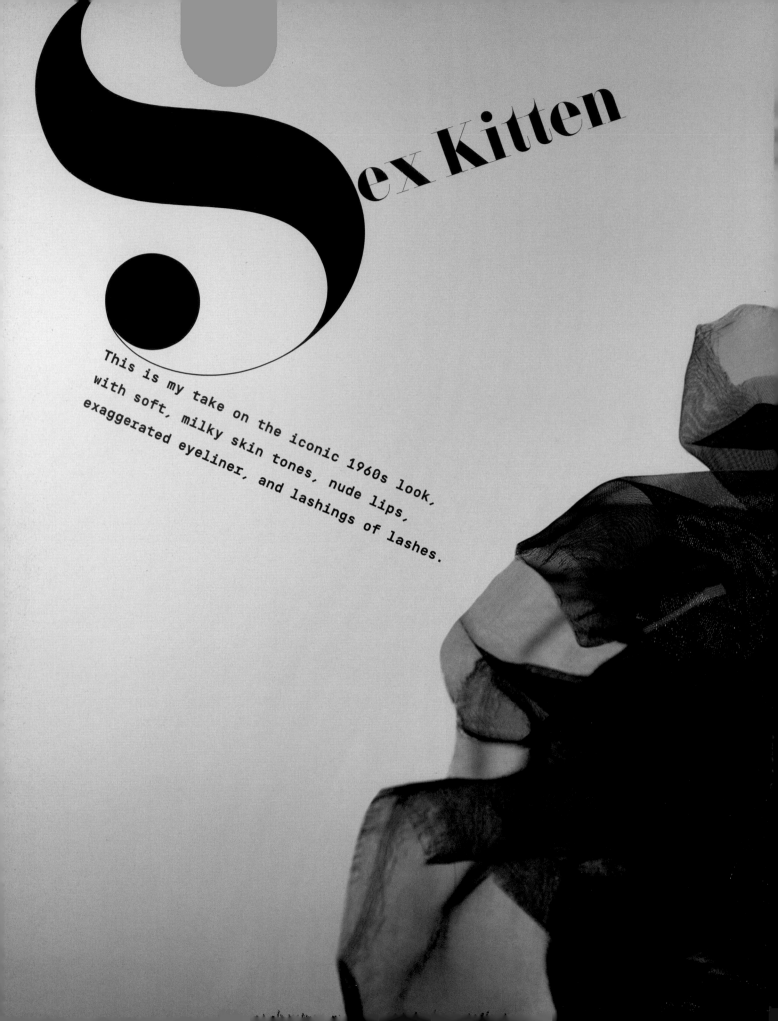

Sex Kitten

This is my take on the iconic 1960s look, with soft, milky skin tones, nude lips, exaggerated eyeliner, and lashings of lashes.

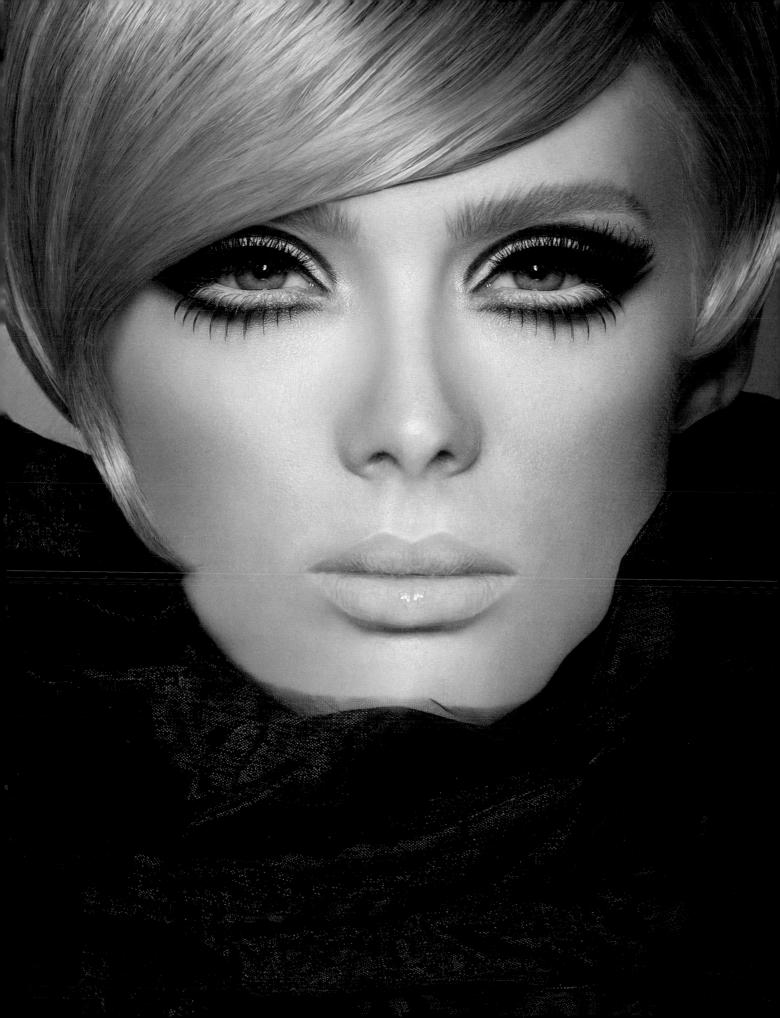

Sex Kitten Transformation

The vivacious, flirtatious glamour epitomized by sex symbols such as Brigitte Bardot and Sophia Loren sums up this look perfectly. I also think of Edie Sedgwick and Twiggy, key players in the Swinging Sixties scene that centered on London's Carnaby Street. It was a revolutionary time, and fashion and make-up were obvious outlets for the newfound freedom of expression. This is a bold, geometric look— all black and white—with the focus on the retro eyeliner, heavy sockets, false lashes galore, and lashings of mascara. Groomed brows, à la Elizabeth Taylor, frame the face, which is creamy and flawless, with sexy lips in matte or glossy pastel pink, peach, or nude. The key to this look is the sharp, flicked-up eyeliner and the dramatic black socket. On our model [previous spread], I left a gap between these elements for an exaggerated doe-eyed look, and finished her lips with creamy pale pink lipstick to flatter her fair complexion. Charlotte's transformation demonstrates a more wearable version of this look, as I blended a little black matte eyeshadow onto the outer corner of the eyes to connect the socket crease and the winged eyeliner, softening and emphasizing the outer edge of the eyes and drawing her eyes apart.

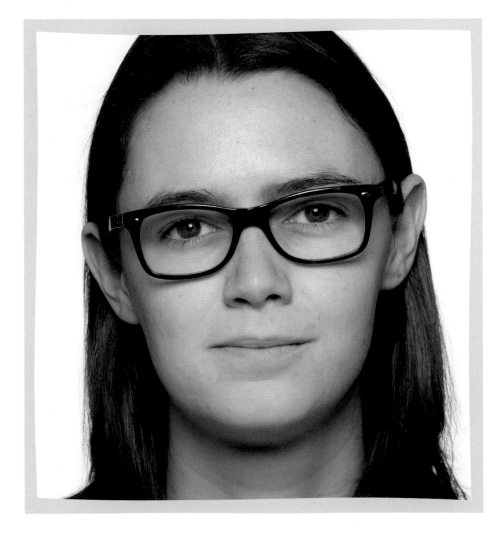

Charlotte, who is in her twenties, doesn't wear much make-up and often wears glasses that hide her pretty eyes. I wanted to show her how to play up this great feature by defining her eyes with an exaggerated feline flick that could easily be made more wearable for everyday (see page 150).

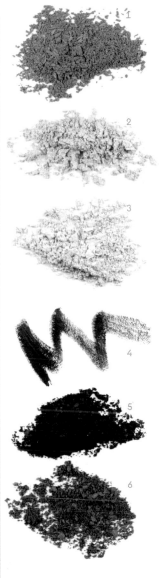

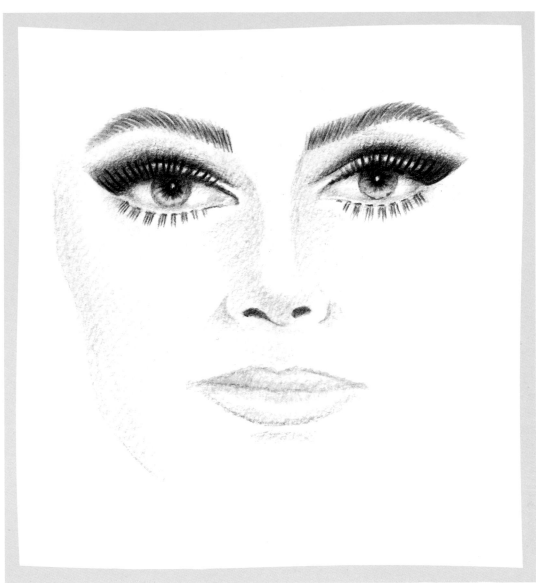

face

Color correctors.
Concealer.
Cream foundation to match
the skin tone.
Darker and lighter shades
of cream foundation for
contouring.
Translucent powder.
Apricot powder blush (1).
Champagne highlighter (2).

eyes

Light brown matte
brow powder.
Warm off-white matte
powder eyeshadow (3).
Black gel eyeliner (4).
Black matte powder
eyeshadow (5).
Charcoal matte powder
eyeshadow (6).
Black mascara.
Two (optional) full strips of
long, doll-like false lashes
(7 and 8).

lips

Nude lip liner with a pinky
peach tone (9).
Creamy nude lipstick with
a satin finish (10).
Clear lip gloss.

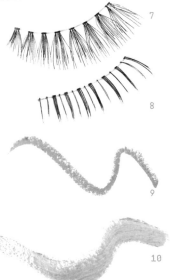

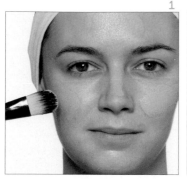

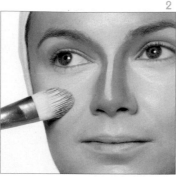

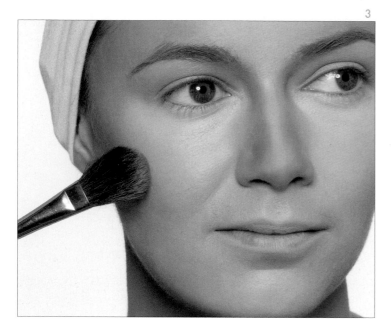

Tip For classic Elizabeth Taylor eyebrows, make the beginning of your brows fuller. Build up the color gradually, graduating the tone slightly from light to dark [see page 97]. Remember not to make the brows too dark, as it will kill the look.

■face

1 After prepping and priming the skin as usual (see pages 28–9), I addressed any blemishes with color correctors and concealer (see pages 30–1), and applied cream foundation all over her face for a flawless complexion.

2 I then used two shades of cream foundation to contour her face. Charlotte has a long, rectangular face, so I wanted to balance this out by creating the illusion of fuller, rounder cheeks. I used the darker shade to soften her temples and jawline, slim down her nose, and create depth around the eye socket and below the cheekbones. Then I applied the lighter color to brighten and highlight under the eyes and other areas that I wanted to bring forward (see pages 56–61).

3 I blended the hard edges with a soft blending brush to create a natural-looking finish and applied a light dusting of translucent powder to set the make-up.

■eyes

4 Having tweezed any stray hairs to create a higher arch, I filled in her brows with a light brown matte brow powder using a soft angled brush. To make the beginning of the brows look thicker, I applied the color onto the skin just under the brow line and blended it onto the arch. To exaggerate the shape, I took the color slightly above the natural arch and blended it down to the outer corner using feathery strokes.

5 To create the illusion of lots of space on the eye, I applied a wash of warm off-white matte eyeshadow all over the lid and up to the brow bone. I then used a small angled brush to apply black gel eyeliner on the upper lash line, winging it out and up at the outer edge of the eye. This look is about exaggerating the line and taking it further than you normally would. It might not feel natural when you're drawing it, but it looks really effective. I went over the line with black matte powder eyeshadow to soften it.

6 Next, I cut out a crease slightly above the natural socket line in charcoal matte powder eyeshadow. I drew this with a small angled brush to create a clean, sharp line. I connected the end of this line with the outer tip of the winged eyeliner and filled in the triangle with the charcoal eyeshadow to emphasize the outer corner of the eye. If you want to create a wider space for a doe-eyed look (as I did on page 153), don't connect the lines together but just taper the eyeshadow to nothing. I slightly softened the inner edge of the triangle, but didn't blend the crease line as I wanted it to remain sharp.

7 I curled the upper lashes and applied a coat of black mascara before adding a full strip of long, doll-like false lashes for that exaggerated 1960s look.

8 To increase the wide-eyed effect, I then applied a strip to the bottom lashes.

9 Finally, I added another coat of mascara to the roots of the upper lashes.

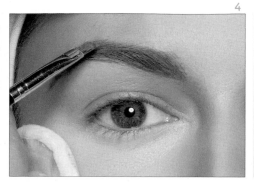

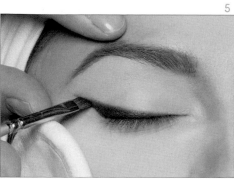

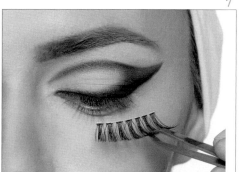

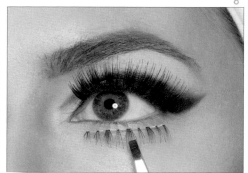

Tip Hold your eyelid taut when you apply the liner to help keep the line straight and smooth.

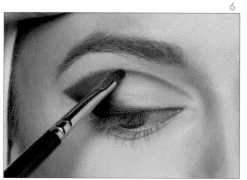

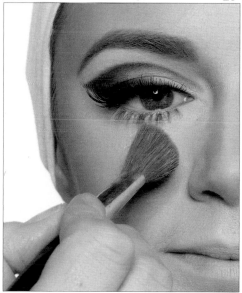

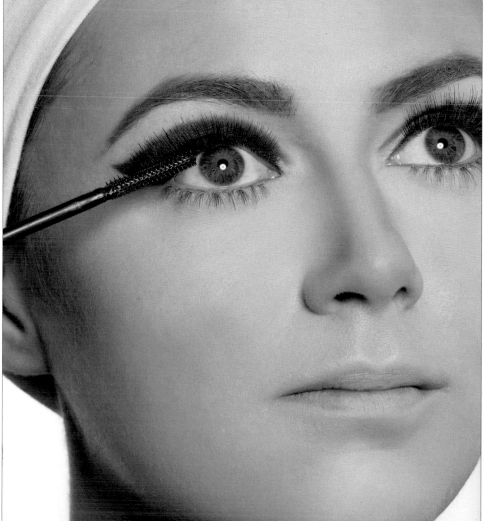

■finish

10 As the eye make-up is so strong, I wanted to soften the face and bring a little extra life to the skin, so I applied a little apricot blush to the cheeks, to add warmth, and a touch of champagne highlighter under the eyes, along the tops of the cheekbones, and on the center of the forehead, chin, and upper lip.

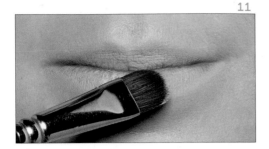

11

■lips

11 All the drama is on the eyes, so I counterbalanced the look with classic nude lips. First, to neutralize the natural pigment in the lips and create a smooth base for the lipstick, I applied a little foundation all over the lips—you can use concealer or primer for this, as long as it matches your skin tone.

12 I outlined the lips with a nude lip pencil with a pinky peach undertone that matched the lipstick, drawing the line just outside the natural lip line to create the illusion of fuller lips. Then I filled in the shape and blotted the lips with a tissue for greater staying power.

13 Using a lip brush, I applied creamy nude lipstick all over the lips.

14 To emphasize the Cupid's bow and make the lips look fuller, I applied a touch of the champagne highlighter above the upper lip.

15 I wanted to make the lips look as full and luscious as possible, so I added a hint of gloss to the middle of the bottom lip.

12

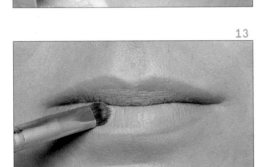

13

14

15

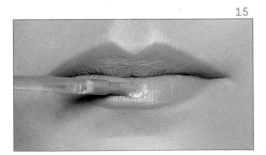

Tips

» This may take a few goes to master; make sure you draw the crease line where it can be seen when your eyes are open.

» Applying a false-lash strip to the bottom lashes is fiddly and does require practice to perfect the technique.

» When using full-strip lashes, be careful not to channel *A Clockwork Orange*—adding individual lashes at the outer edge gives a softer finish that may suit you better.

» Lip liner is not essential for this look but it will give the lips extra definition and make the lipstick last longer.

» A nude matte lipstick also looks great with this look, but a glossy finish will make the lips appear fuller.

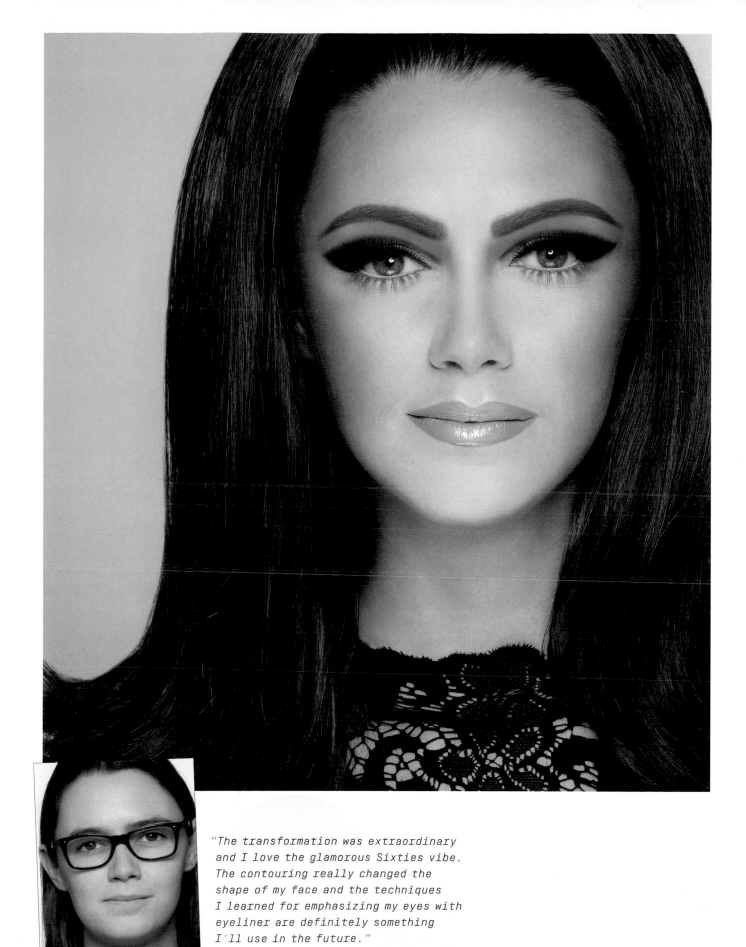

"The transformation was extraordinary
and I love the glamorous Sixties vibe.
The contouring really changed the
shape of my face and the techniques
I learned for emphasizing my eyes with
eyeliner are definitely something
I'll use in the future."

Perfect glamorous eye

One of the most effective ways to accentuate the eyes is to contour them by cutting out a crease and creating areas of light and shadow, framed by a beautifully defined lash line and fluttery lashes. This is achieved using three graduating tones of eyeshadow, as well as eyeliner, false lashes, and mascara. The lightest shade of eyeshadow is blended over the first three-quarters of the lid and under the brow bone, the mid-tone is swept into the crease and outer corner, and the darkest tone is used to soften the eyeliner and create more depth at the outer corner. This technique has the effect of deepening the socket, elongating the eyes, pulling them apart, and lifting the outer corners.

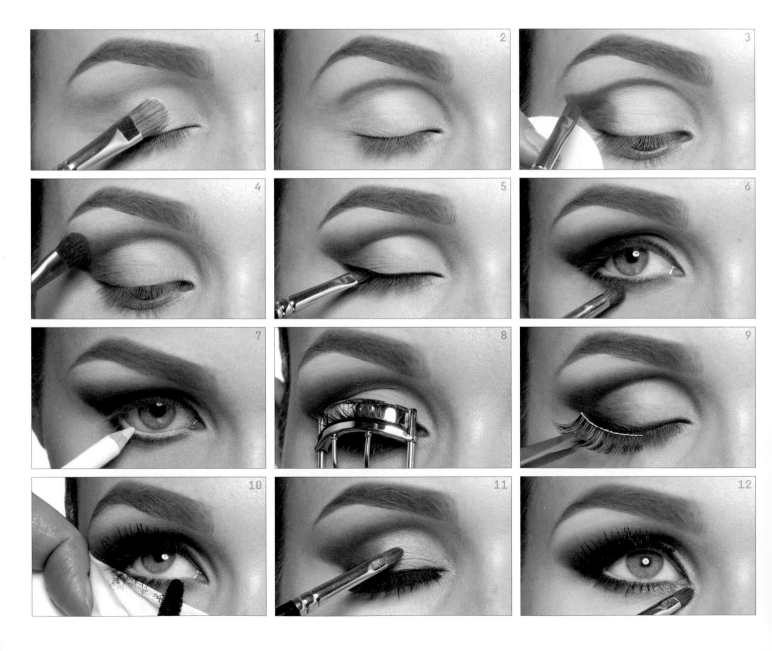

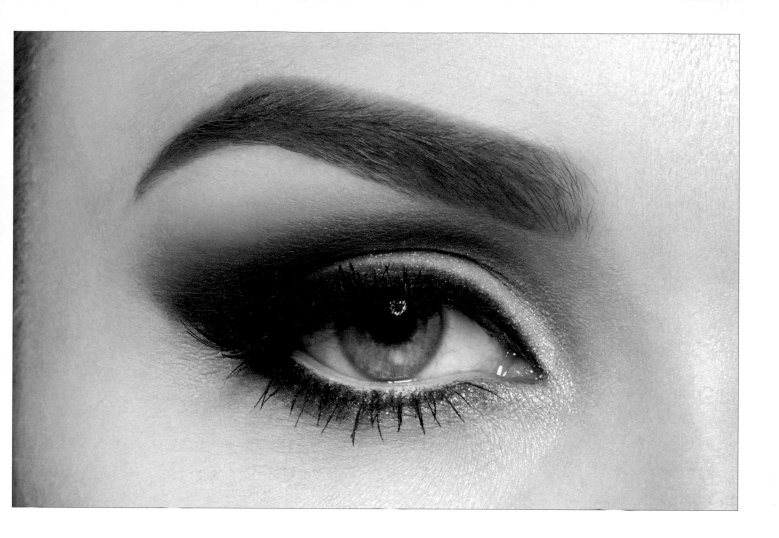

1 Create a beautifully tailored brow to frame the look (see page 97). Then, with a mid-sized flat eyeshadow brush, apply bone-colored matte eyeshadow across the lid and under the brow bone to open up the area and make it look bigger.

2 Cut out a crease with a mid-brown shade. Work it into the socket line, taking it slightly higher than the natural socket to give the illusion of a bigger eye with a higher, deeper socket. Do this looking straight into the mirror with your eyes open to ensure you get the crease in the correct place. Use an angled brush to create a sharper line or a pencil brush for a softer effect.

3 With an angled brush, extend the socket line out and down toward the outer corner of the eye. Take the color up from the lash line at the outer corner, sweeping it up and out to meet the end of the socket line, creating a triangle shape. Fill in this section to elongate and lift the eye.

4 Using a soft brush, blend the color into the lighter color on the lid and soften all the edges. Make sure you don't take the color too low, as the aim is to lift the outer corners.

5 Apply black or dark brown gel or cream eyeliner with a small angled brush. The line should start off thin at the beginning of the eye, becoming thicker and lifting up slightly at the outer edge to follow the line created with the eyeshadow.

6 With a pencil brush, apply dark brown eyeshadow under the eye, blending it into the outer corner and onto the upper lash line to soften the eyeliner.

7 To give the eyes that sparkly, wide-awake look, apply a nude-toned eyeliner on the waterline. If you have large or protruding eyes, use a dark brown eyeliner; if you want a really sultry effect, use a black pencil eyeliner.

8 Curl the lashes to open up the eye.

9 Add a fluttery strip lash or lash clusters to enhance your eye shape (see page 136–9).

10 Holding a tissue under your lashes to prevent smudges, coat the bottom lashes with mascara. If you've applied false lashes, just concentrate on the roots to add volume.

11–12 Finish off the look with an accent of shimmer to catch the light and bring the eyes alive. Choose a vanilla pigment that complements the tones of the eyeshadows used, and add a touch to the middle of the lid and around the tear duct.

Balance this glamorous, sexy eye with a creamy or glossy lipstick in a neutral taupe.

Favorite eye looks

With so many eyeshadows in wonderful hues and textures, not to mention amazing pigments, eyeliners, mascaras, and false eyelashes, it's easy to create dramatically different looks to suit the occasion and your mood. From a sheer colorwash or a natural and nude eye for daytime or to complement a strong lip, to a glamorous contoured eye or a statement flick, there are almost endless ways to make up the eyes. Here are some of my favorites.

1 neutral This sumptuous eye, framed by a full, groomed brow, features chocolate eyeshadow fed into the socket, swept under the eye, and softly blended—perfect for accentuating green or hazel eyes.

2 soft flick This soft feline flick is top heavy, with nothing under the eye, and vanilla eyeshadow on the lid with a slightly darker tone in the socket. Corner lashes draw attention to the outer edge of the eye.

3 sexy smoky For this dark, sultry eye, the waterlines are rimmed with kohl, and charcoal eyeshadow is blended all over the lid and under the eyes to create maximum drama.

4 vibrant A natural brow lets the bright hues take center stage. Shimmery violets look great on skin with cool undertones.

5 contoured This glamorous, elongated eye is all about the color gradient, with the darkest shade at the corner, the mid-tone in the middle, and the lightest at the beginning of the eye.

6 metallic For a high-shine evening look, silver cream eyeshadow is made more wearable by blending brown eyeshadow into the socket.

7 glitter Perfect for parties, gold and turquoise hues combined with electric-blue liner and mascara are brought to life with high-shine pigment and sparkly glitter.

8 soft smoky Toning shades of burgundy and mocha eyeshadows are blended softly to create a smoky eye for daytime or evening.

9 vintage flick The sexy, exaggerated flick and corner lashes lengthen and lift the eye—perfect for anyone with round or close-set eyes.

10 colorwash A wash of color—in cream or powder, shimmer or matte—is an easy daytime look. Just curl the lashes and add mascara.

11 bronzed Shimmering tones of gold and bronze blended over the lids make the eyes pop, with kohl-rimmed waterlines for definition.

12 dramatic flick This statement flick starts off thin and gradually thickens as it lifts up at the corner of the eye. Kohl lining the waterlines intensifies this bold look.

13 wet-look smoky This is a fun but high-maintenance evening look, with a blend of dark cream eyeshadows, kohl pencil, and petroleum jelly for a watery finish.

14 natural The sheer wash of skin-tone shadow—matte or shimmer—is blended over the lid and under the eye for a simple daytime look.

15 classic Neutral tones with a slight shimmer softly contour the eye, while darker tones around the lash line add depth and frame it.

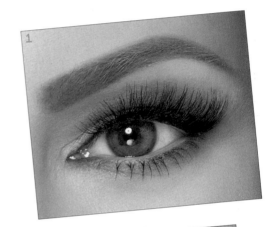

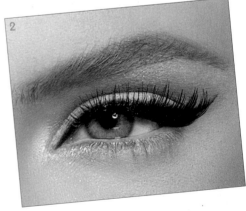

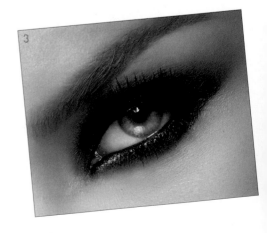

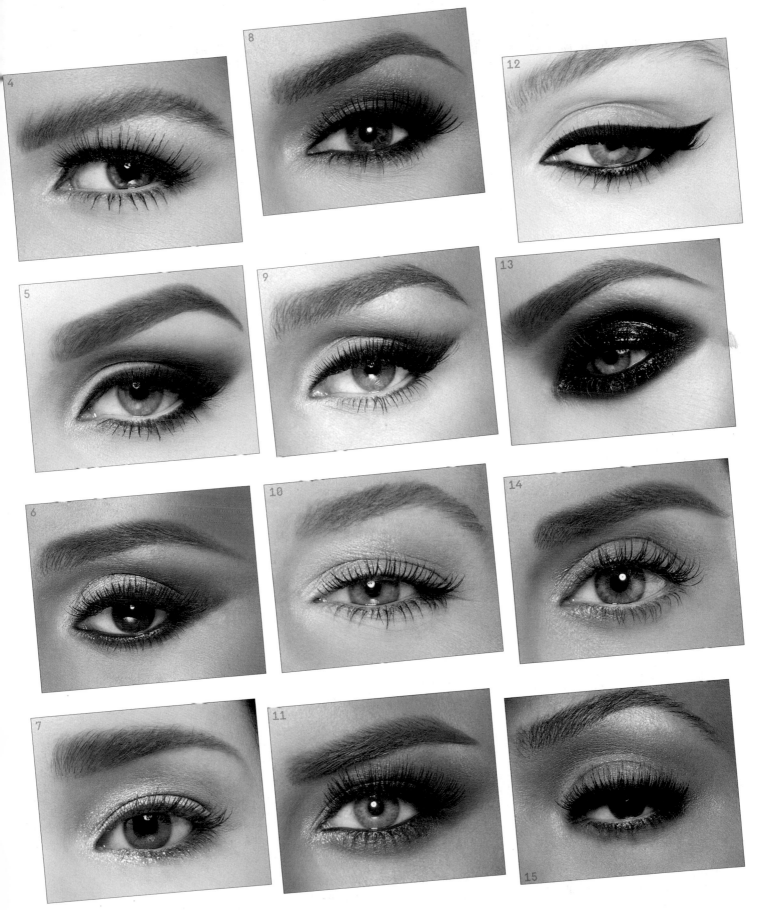

lips

The lips are often
what people focus
on when others talk
or laugh, and they are
a lovely feature to
enhance. You may want
to emphasize both your
eyes and your lips,
or let the lips take
center stage with a
bold bright pink or
orange, a dramatic
deep berry or a sexy
classic scarlet, or
let them play second
fiddle to statement
eyes, in subtle sheer
or creamy nudes. Keep
them well moisturized
and conditioned for
a perfect pout.

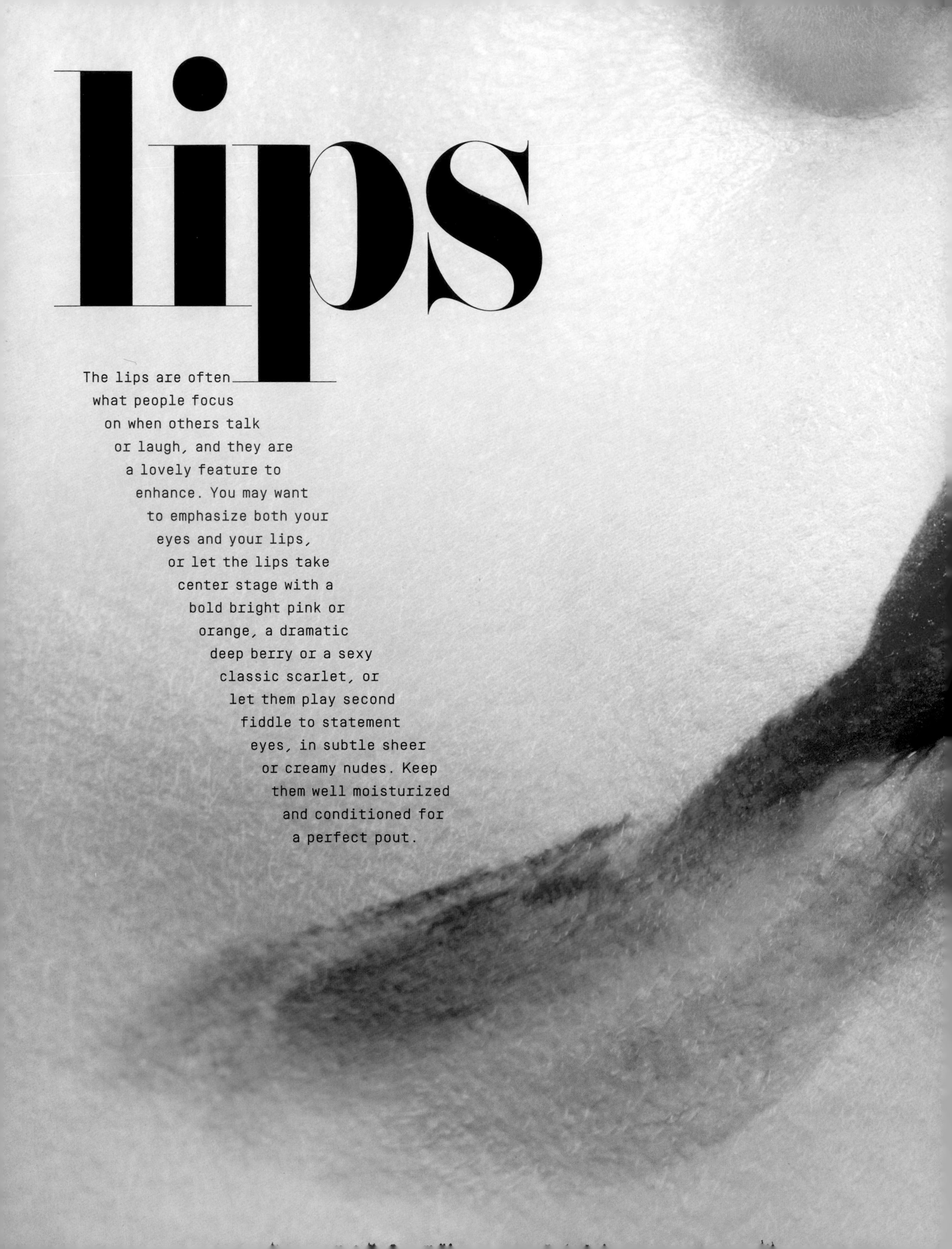

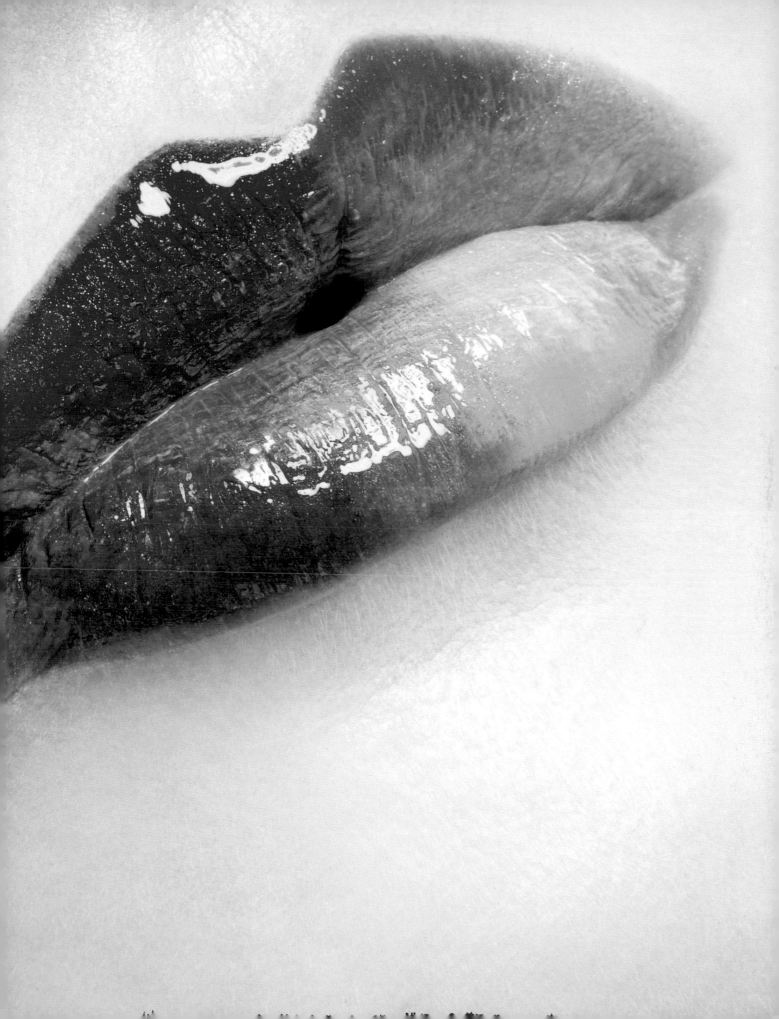

ip shapes

Everyone's lip shape is different and lips are rarely completely symmetrical. So if, like most people, you don't have a perfect pout, here's how to trick everyone into thinking you do. Whether your lips are uneven, too thin, or bottom heavy, the key word is balance. The aim is to achieve a full, symmetrical shape with a defined Cupid's bow.

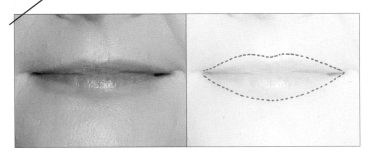

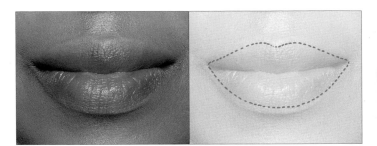

thin lips To make the lips look fuller, the aim is to increase the size of the upper and lower lips and give them a softly curving outline. Apply foundation or concealer, then slightly overline the natural lip shape before filling them in with a pale lipstick in a satin, metallic, or glossy texture. If one lip is thinner than the other, try to even them out.

full lips Most people would love to have full lips, but if you want to play your lips down and make them look less prominent, keep the lipstick inside the natural lip line. Apply concealer or foundation around the outline and draw a new lip line slightly inside the natural line, or don't line the lips at all. Choose a neutral lipstick and a finish that isn't too glossy.

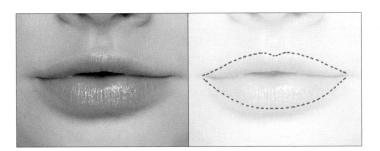

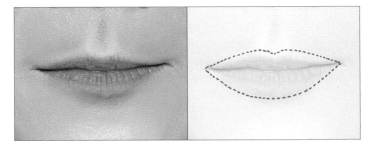

bottom-heavy lips Build up the top lip and play down the bottom lip to create a balanced effect. Slightly overline the top lip and underline the bottom lip, and use a lighter tone on the top lip and a darker one on the bottom lip to make it recede. Apply highlighter above the Cupid's bow and don't use a light-reflective finish on the bottom lip.

flat lips Build up and contour the lips to create more dimension. Use lip liner to draw a Cupid's bow, curving down to the corners of the mouth. Overline the bottom lip to make it look fuller. Keep dark tones to the outer edge of the lips, getting gradually lighter to create fullness; add shimmer or gloss to make the lips look plumper.

Remember:
Dark colors and matte textures make the lips recede and look smaller; light colors and metallic, satin, or glossy textures reflect the light, bring the lips forward and make them look fuller.

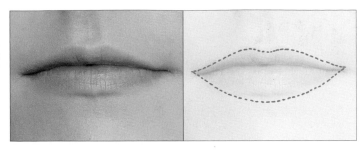

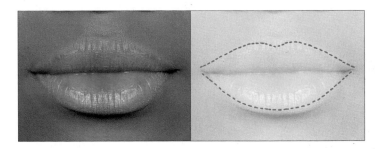

down-turned lips To lift the corners of the mouth, first use foundation to cover the existing lip line. Draw in the Cupid's bow and curve the line down, but stop before you get to the point where the lip turns down. Line the bottom lip, taking it up a little before the corners so it appears to meet the point where the lip liner ends on the upper lip.

round Try to give the mouth more width and the lips more shape. Define the Cupid's bow but draw slightly inside the natural line. Take the lines down to the corners, keeping them slightly straighter rather than curved. Make the top lip slightly darker and matte, and the bottom lip lighter. Avoid any gloss or shimmer toward the outer edges of the mouth.

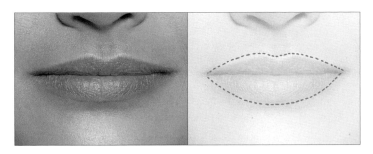

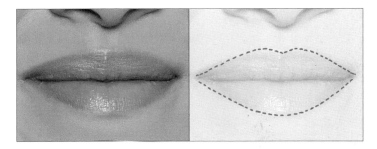

sharp and defined lips Aim to soften the edges and create curves and fullness. Cover the natural lip line with foundation and either don't line the lips or use a matte pencil to create a curved outline, breaking the line slightly and blending it so it's not too defined and hard. A sheer or natural finish will soften and play down the lips.

oval Make more of the Cupid's bow to give the upper lip shape and height. Use lip liner to draw a nice V-shape, then take the line down toward the corners to create more of an angle, keeping both sides symmetrical. To reduce the width of the mouth, don't take the liner all the way to the corners. Highlight the central part of the lips.

key kit

» Foundation, concealer, primer, or powder—to cover the natural shape so you can create a new one. Apply this first.

» Creamy matte lip pencil—to enhance an existing lip line, create a new one, and prevent lipstick from bleeding.

» Lipstick—to enhance the lips.

» Gloss—a touch of clear gloss complements most lips and gives a shiny 3-D effect.

» Highlighter—a dab above or below the lips draws attention and light to the area.

» Tissues—for blotting after each application to help stain the lips and make the lipstick last longer.

» Lip brush—for precision and control, a must when you're correcting the lip shape.

dos and don'ts for aging lips

» Do use foundation or primer on your lips to fill in any grooves or lines.

» Do use a creamy lip liner to prevent the lipstick from bleeding into fine lines around the mouth.

» Do blot with a tissue a few times so the lip liner stains the lips and acts like a barrier before you apply lipstick.

» Do choose a lipstick with a light sheen, as it will be more flattering than a matte finish, which can be harsh and aging.

» If your lips are small, do go for lighter colors, or, if you want to wear red or another deep color, slightly overline the lips to make them look fuller.

» Don't go mad with gloss, as it will travel.

Lip textures and finishes

Lips have never looked better, with all the fabulous formulations that are moisturizing, hydrating, plumping, or long-lasting. Whether you want a youthful berry-red stain, a neutral sheer, a dramatic watery metallic, or a sexy glossy pout, there's something for everyone.

Remember:
By combining textures and color, it's possible to give the lips more dimension and create a fuller, 3-D effect.

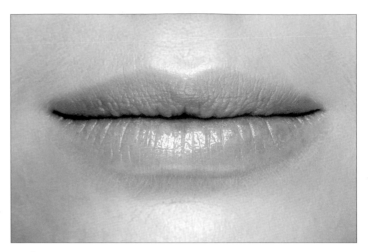

sheer

This is a light formulation that creates a natural finish and is usually very hydrating and moisturizing. Sheer lipstick is easy to apply, suits all ages, and is a great choice for daytime. Tinted lip balms are also very conditioning and give a sheer finish. Even without lip liner, they can make lips look fuller.

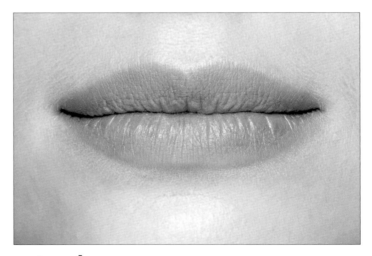

stain

Quick-drying stains are long-lasting and often smudge-proof, but they can dry out the lips. Also, there isn't such a variety of colors to choose from as with other lipsticks. You can create a stain as follows: line the lips with a pencil lip liner, blot with a tissue, apply lipstick, blot, and repeat.

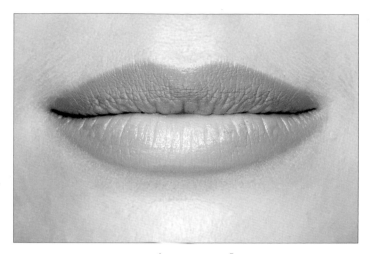

cream/satin

Popular cream or satin lipsticks are very smooth on application and highly moisturizing, giving a rich, shiny, weightless finish that makes the lips look fuller and more luscious. You will need to reapply, especially if you're eating or drinking, but a matte lip liner will help it stay in place for longer and minimize bleeding. A great choice for older lips.

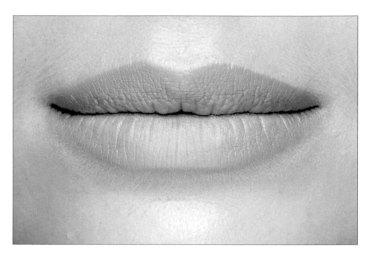

matte

For depth, drama, and full coverage, nothing beats matte lipstick. It gives a really rich, velvety, opaque, and long-lasting finish. The flat color is less likely to bleed but it can be drying. To counteract this, apply a little moisturizer or primer to the lips and then blot with a tissue before applying matte lipstick.

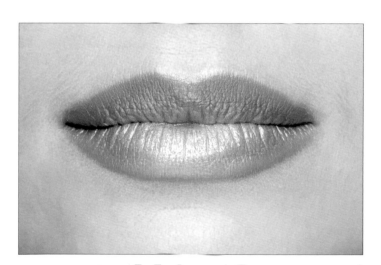

metallic/frosted

With its high-shine finish, metallic or frosted lipstick is something you would probably wear more in the evening. Metallic lipstick is highly pigmented and light-reflective, so it gives a luxurious, pearlized finish with a good color pay-off. It comes in a wide choice of colors, and while it's not as wearable as some of the other textures, it's great for a party.

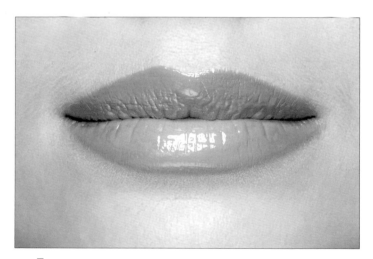

gloss

Clear or colored, glittery, or metallic, lip gloss gives that watery, high-impact shine that can look fantastic, but horrendous if it's not used correctly—apply only a dab to the center of the bottom lip. It's the most high-maintenance of all lip textures and can highlight a thin lip, making it look thinner and uneven. Petroleum jelly will give a similar effect.

How to wear Color

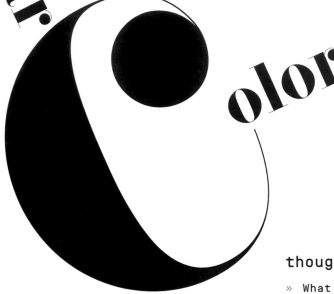

There's nothing like a splash of color on the lips to lift the mood and transform the face. There are so many bold, beautiful hues and wonderful formulations to choose from, whether you favor a natural or a statement look, the sheerest hint of soft color or vibrant, saturated tones. The lips are a great place to showcase color—most people feel more comfortable wearing bold colors on their lips than on their eyes—and lipsticks are a great way to express your personality. They say a lot about your mood—whether you're feeling sexy, confident, outgoing, wholesome, or sensual.

Choosing lipsticks and glosses doesn't have to be complex—anything goes, as long as it's flattering and you feel good in it. Some people choose their lipstick to go with their clothes, but I think picking an accent color from your outfit and matching your lipstick to that—perhaps the color of your purse or shoes—is more dynamic and interesting.

Fashion and trends can sometimes influence the popularity of a lipstick color or texture, and it's often instinctive to change your lipstick with the seasons. Those mouthwatering bright oranges and corals seem right in the summer months, while more muted tones, neutrals, and berry shades feel safer in the winter.

Don't underestimate the power of color on the lips. It can work with very minimal make-up on the rest of the face and look amazing, but if you have great eyes as well as great lips, and your face can take it, there's no reason why you can't pair bright lips with bold eyes.

thoughts on lip color

» What works on fair skin may not suit dark skin, and vice versa.

» For warm skin tones, try browns, oranges, nudes, taupes, golds, and caramels.

» For cool skin tones, try shades of pink, peach, and purple.

» Pale lipstick makes lips look fuller.

» Darker shades and matte textures make lips look thinner, so overline them slightly.

» A matte finish will make a bright or deep color look more extreme, as the color is denser.

» A touch of gloss makes a color softer and the lips more 3-D.

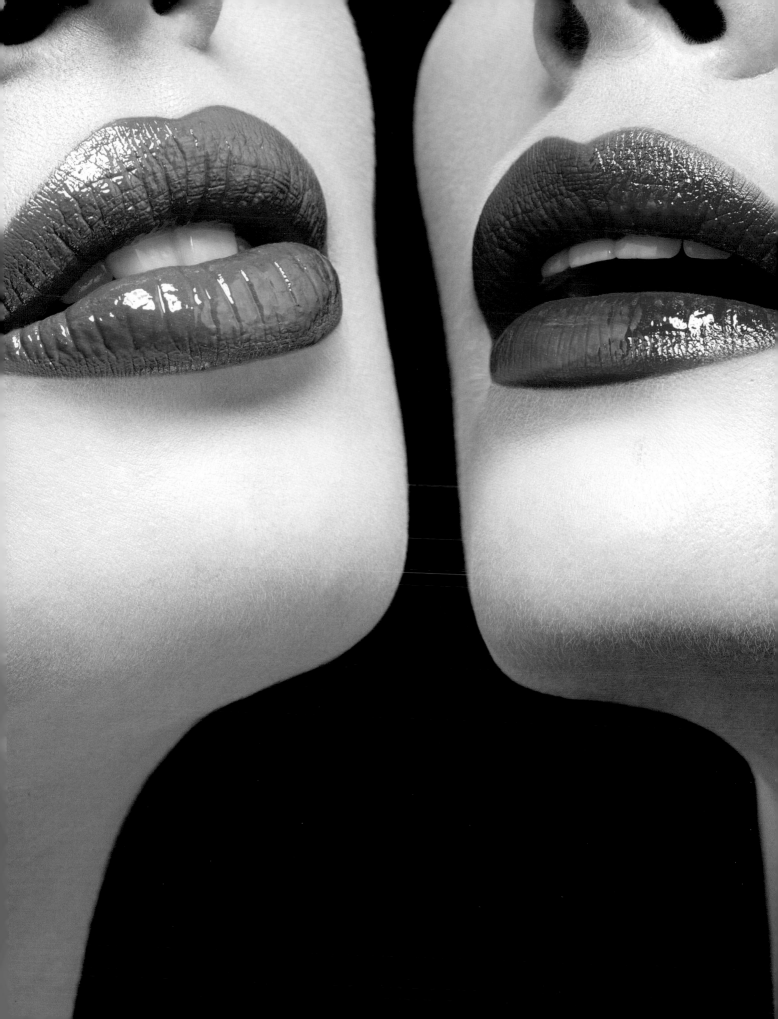

favorite lip colors

Whether you're wanting to play up your lips, your eyes, or both, choose your lipstick color and finish in relation to your whole look, to ensure all the tones and textures work together. Bold and bright, deep and dramatic, or nude and natural, there's a shade that will work with your skin tone and hair coloring. Here are some of my favorites.

1 glossy pink nude This sumptuous, creamy, pinky beige lipstick has been finished with gloss to create sexy, full, evening lips.

2 burnt-orange satin This is a great summertime color for mid-toned skin, bringing a soft, sexy warmth to the face.

3 metallic bronze This bronze metallic lip gloss reflects the light and is great for creating full lips that work well with shimmering warm tones.

4 glamorous nude These flesh-toned lips are contoured with a darker shade on the outer edge and a lighter one in the middle to create fullness, with gloss to emphasize the Cupid's bow.

5 sheer gloss This shimmering, gold-toned gloss draws attention to the mouth without the need for lip liner and can be worn day or night.

6 red satin Classic red lips are suitable for the day or evening. A satin finish is flattering for older or smaller mouths, and matching lip liner gives a neat outline and prevents bleeding.

7 daytime nude The lips have been lined and filled in with a soft apricot lip liner and layered with a rich, creamy lipstick. A touch of gloss adds fullness to the lower lip.

8 dark berry drama A deep berry lipstick makes a statement on fair skin but is also flattering on darker skin tones. It looks striking matte, but the high-maintenance glossy finish adds richness and impact.

9 classic claret A creamy, rich claret lipstick, matching lip pencil, and clear lip gloss were used for this stunning evening look. The gloss on the bottom lip reflects the light and makes it come forward and look fuller.

10 fuchsia gloss Vibrant fuchsia lips make a bold, bright statement. The creamy lipstick gives full coverage, and gloss increases the impact.

11 sheer nude An understated pale pink lip balm creates sheer nude lips for a soft, natural look. It's great for the daytime but also works well at night paired with dramatic eyes.

12 pinky red A satin red lipstick with a pink undertone looks great on cool-toned skin for day or evening.

13 peach tint A soft peach multipurpose tint that can also be worn on the cheeks and eyes gives lips a fresh, low-maintenance daytime look.

14 mocha Rich tones of mocha and caramel with a shiny satin finish look gorgeous on darker skin tones. Lined with a creamy pencil, this makes a sexy evening or daytime look.

15 matte red For a bold daytime statement or red-carpet evening glamour, nothing beats timeless scarlet lips—but the matte texture wouldn't look good on older lips.

16 opaque nude These contoured pale nude lips—darker on the edges and lighter in the middle—have a pearlized finish for a perfect full pout.

17 coral and gold Creamy coral lipstick has been topped with gold pigment in the center to create dimension, depth, and fullness. Shiny pigment is a great alternative to gloss.

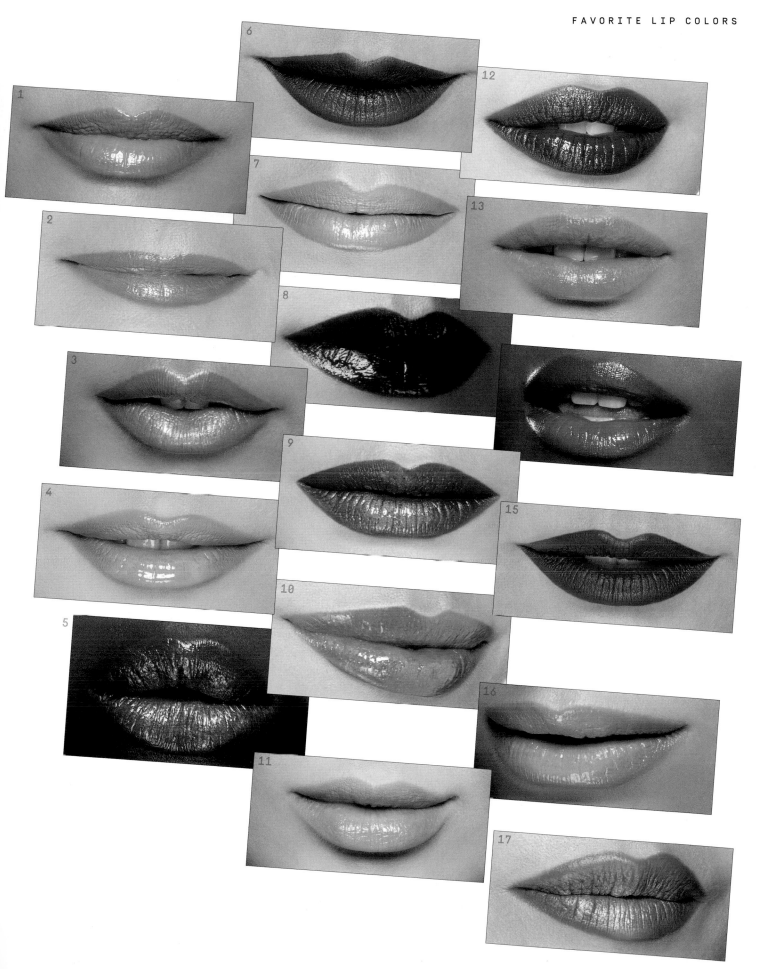

Fairy tale

Bewitching, sublime, and alluring, this is a look that would enchant any handsome prince and put him under your spell.

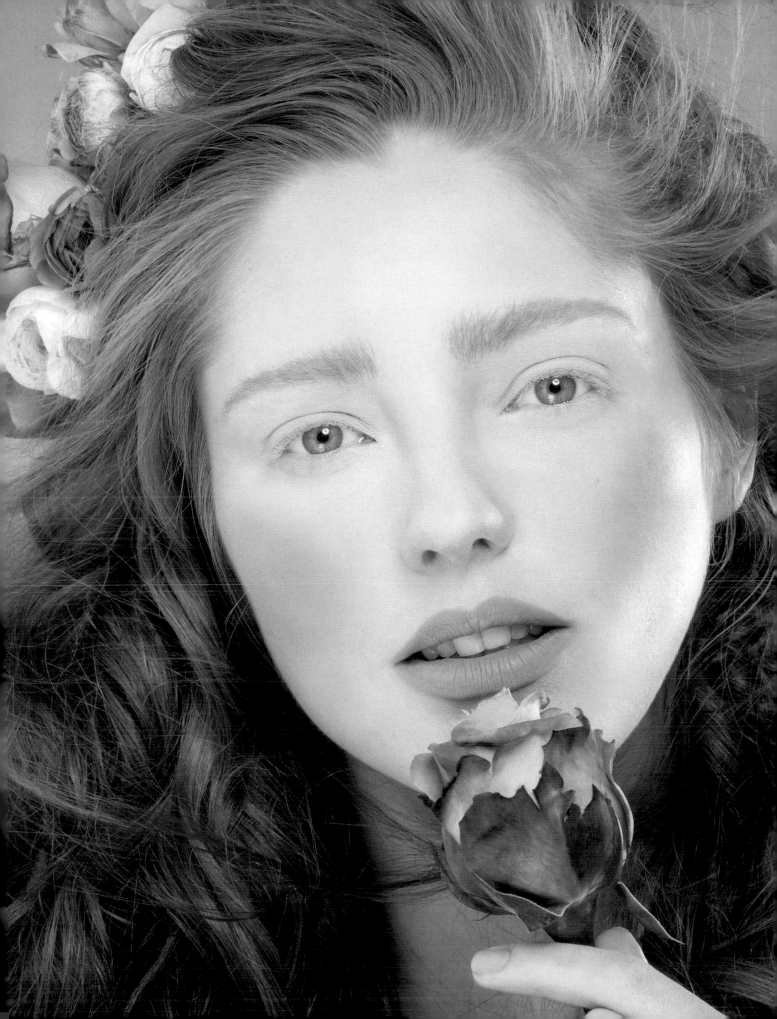

Fairy-Tale Transformation

This ultra-feminine look conjures up romantic florals and blossom-heavy boughs in summer gardens. A take on the classic "English rose" make-up, it's pretty, innocent, youthful, and fresh, with a palette of peaches and cream, rose-petal reds, and pastel pinks and lilacs in creamy, sheer, or shimmering textures. The skin is clear and radiant and the eyes are kept neutral in iridescent oyster, pearl, or apricot, or a soft pastel if you want to introduce some color. All the focus is on the cheeks and lips, which are accentuated with rosy tints and berry stains. Anyone can wear this understated look; the key is to use light-reflecting, hydrating finishes to illuminate the complexion. Choose an eyeshadow with a slight sheen but avoid frosted finishes. Steer clear of cooler toned pastels on older skin, sticking to neutrals and peach or apricot. Our flame-haired model [previous page] looks stunning with pastel-pink lips, rose-dusted cheeks, and powder-blue eyes, like a modern-day pre-Raphaelite painting. For the transformation on Mary, I wanted her young skin to be glowing and dewy, her cheeks accented with rose-pink cream blush, and her lips classic and berry-stained. With her wild hair and mischievous smile, she looks like a beautiful, ethereal woodland nymph.

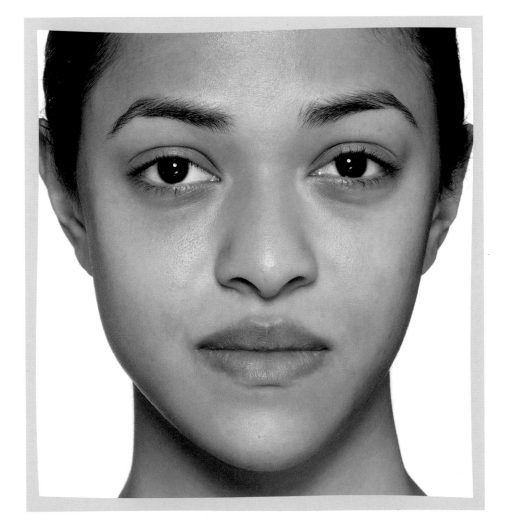

Mary is in her early twenties and I thought this look would really enhance her beautiful skin. The last thing I wanted to do was put too much make-up on her face—you're only young once and should celebrate it and make the most of your youthful looks while you can.

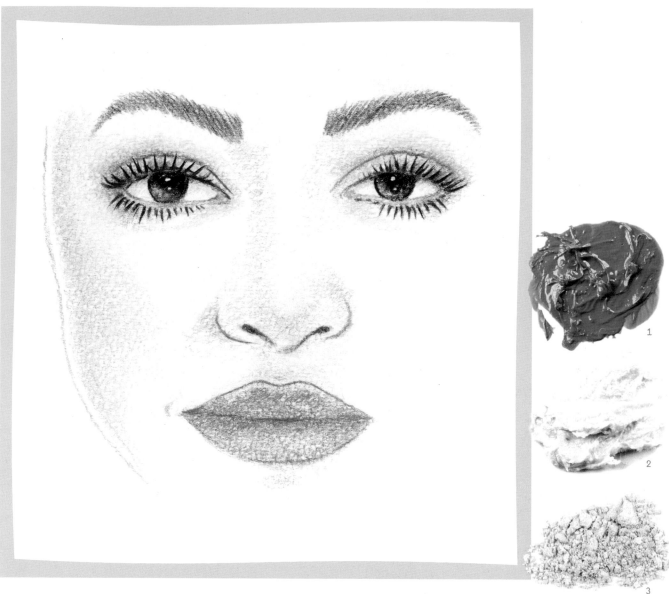

face
Color correctors.
CC cream to match the
skin tone.
Translucent powder.
Rose-pink cream blush (1).
Cream highlighter (2).

eyes
Light brown matte
brow powder.
Slightly pearlized, oyster
powder eyeshadow (3).
Black mascara.
Mid-brown or black gel
eyeliner (4).
Individual false lashes (5).

lips
Soft rose lipstick (6).

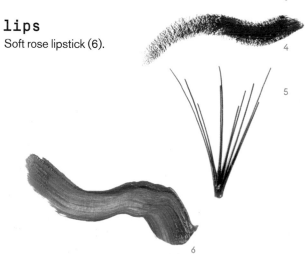

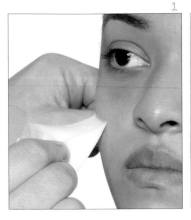

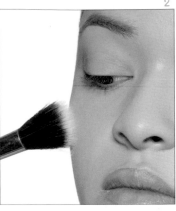

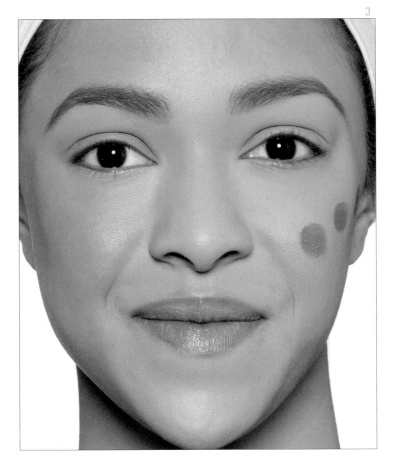

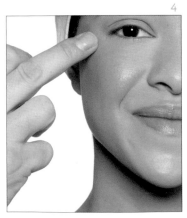

■face

1 Mary has beautiful skin, which I didn't want to cover up. After prepping and priming (see pages 28–9), I addressed any blemishes with color correctors and then applied a touch of CC cream, which has a light, dewy finish but enough coverage to even out her skin tone.

2 I set this with a very light dusting of translucent powder in the areas that I felt needed it.

3 I dabbed a rose-pink cream blush onto the apples of her cheeks and blended it up onto her cheekbones with my fingertip to create a rosy flush. You can do this with a brush, if you prefer, but the warmth of your finger can help to move the cream around on your cheek.

4 I added a little cream highlighter onto the top of her cheekbones and any other area that I wanted to catch the light.

■eyes

5 I brushed up her eyebrows and filled in any gaps with a small angled brush and light brown matte brow powder, following the line of her arch to keep them very natural.

6 I used a slightly pearlized oyster powder eyeshadow and applied it as a wash over the whole lid and eye space, working it right into the socket and blending it softly up to the brow bone.

7 I curled the upper lashes (see page 134) for a wide-eyed innocent look.

8 Because Mary's hair is dark, I applied black mascara to the top and bottom lashes, using a tissue to protect the cheek from smudges. If you are fair, dark brown mascara will give a softer finish.

9 With a small angled brush, I applied a fine, soft line of mid-brown gel eyeliner just above the lash line, pushing the color right into the roots of the lashes. This creates depth and the impression of a shadow above the lash line.

10 For a very natural fluttery effect, I applied a few individual false lashes (see page 139) at the outer edge of her upper lash line.

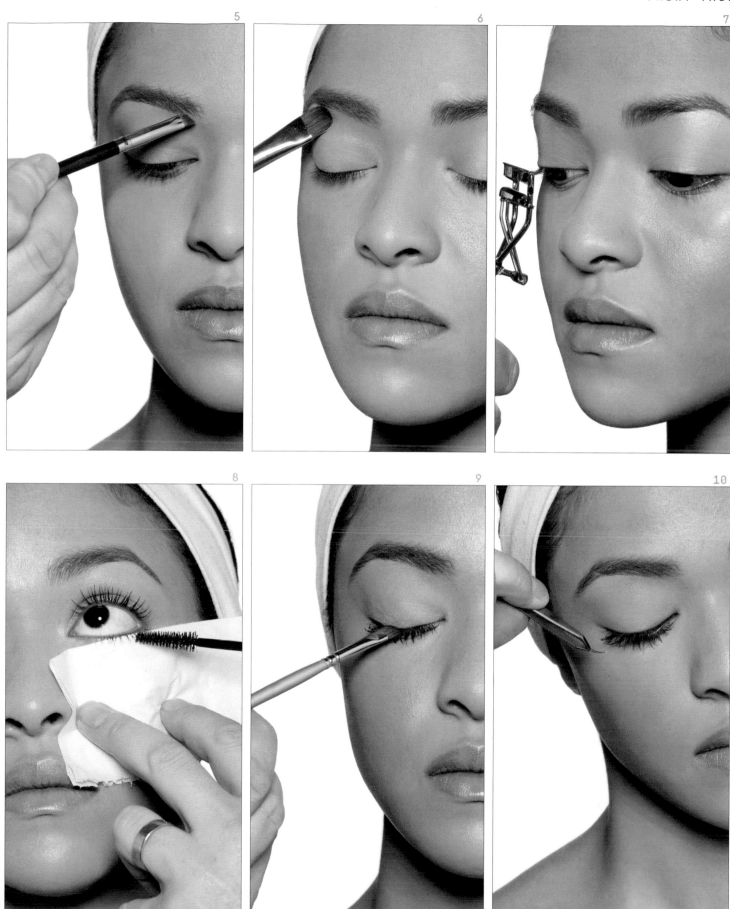

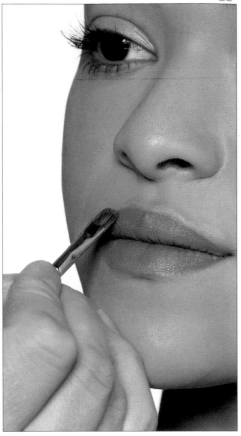

■lips

11 I finished the lips with a soft rose lipstick—no liner, just a simple wash of color that can be sheer, stain, matte, or have a slight shimmer.

Tips

» Choose an eyeshadow with a slight sheen or shimmer that will reflect the light, but steer clear of frosted eyeshadows.

» If you want to use a color on the eyes, go for a soft pastel wash but nothing too strong.

» If you want to keep it neutral, choose pearl, oyster, or apricot eyeshadow with a slight sheen.

» Tidy the eyebrows, brush them up, and fill in any gaps, but keep them very natural.

» If you want to add lashes to give your eyes more definition, go for fine individual lashes in the outer corners.

» Both the cheeks and lips look great with a youthful stain or a sheer finish with a slight shimmer.

» Red, bee-stung lips, which can be done with a matte stain, will make more of a statement.

» To find the color of the natural pigment in your lips and cheeks, pinch your cheek and gently bite your lips—that's the tone of blush and lipstick you should choose for a natural look.

Remember: Create a stain on your lips by blotting them with a tissue between applications of lip liner and lipstick.

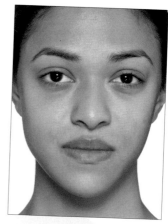

"I love the freshness of this low-key, romantic look and I think it's something I could re-create quite easily now that I've seen how it's done. My skin looks radiant and glowing and I loved the pretty rosy lip stain."

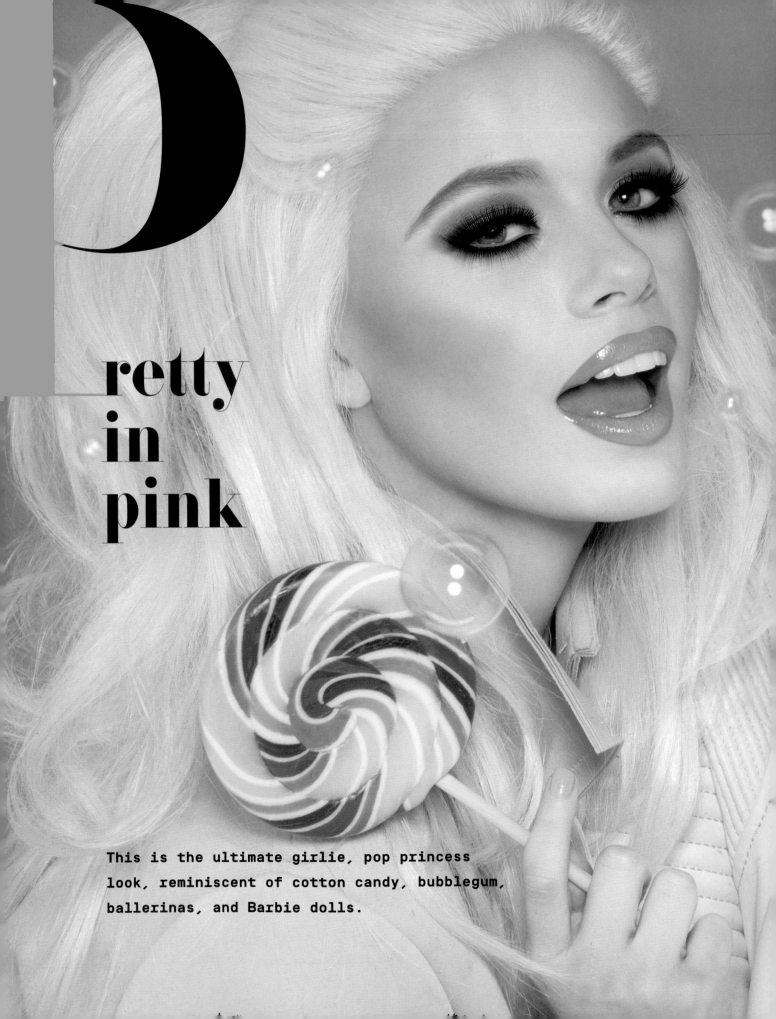

Pretty in pink

This is the ultimate girlie, pop princess look, reminiscent of cotton candy, bubblegum, ballerinas, and Barbie dolls.

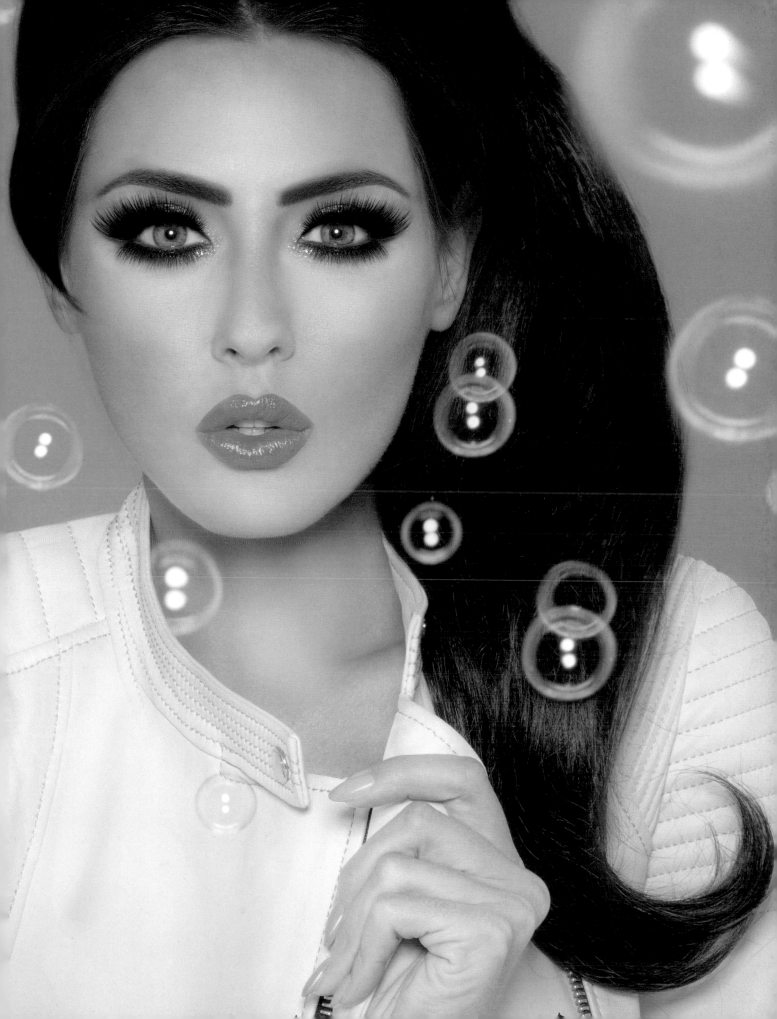

Pretty in Pink Transformation

This exaggerated look is all about playing around with bold, bright pinks and purples to emphasize both the eyes and lips. More is definitely more, so take the look to the max for the full-on color-pop effect. Think of 1950s diners and experiment with ice-cream shades of violet cream, blueberry muffin, strawberry milkshake, and sugar frosting. On our models [previous spread], I wanted to take the make-up to the extreme for a plastic-fantastic, doll-like, cartoon effect. After working on their skin to make it creamy and flawless, I added lots of color to their faces with clashing pinks, purples, and blues, and

finished the look with over-the-top lashes, top and bottom. This make-up is for girls who want to have fun, so give the exhibitionist in you free rein to indulge in some splashy candy colors. You don't want to resemble a drag queen, but if you've got the features and the confidence to carry it off, then go for it. For the transformation on Tamara, I wanted to make the most of her full lips with playful, eye-popping fuchsia lipstick, offset by gorgeous, girlie pink and lilac eyes. Even though I used a lot of bold colors and false lashes, the coverage on her skin is light and radiant, so the result is young, fresh, and fun.

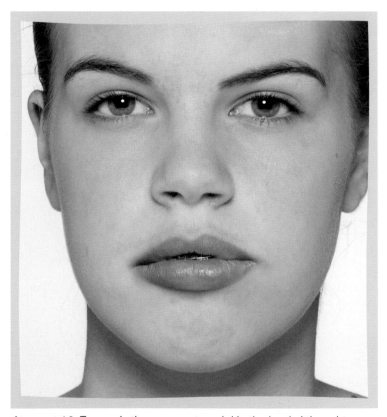

At sweet 16, Tamara is the youngest model in the book. I thought she'd be perfect for this look, as she loves make-up and her favorite color is pink. When you're a teenager, it's a great time to experiment with color, and this fun look shows how to take it to the max with bold, bright hues.

face
Color correctors.
Tinted moisturizer to match the skin tone.
Translucent powder.
Candy-pink blush (1).
Highlighter (2).

eyes
Light ash-blonde matte brow powder.
Vanilla pigment (3).
Shimmery cotton-candy-pink powder eyeshadow (4).
Hot-pink powder eyeshadow (5).
Black gel eyeliner (6).
Black mascara.
Feathery strip of false lashes (7).
Black matte powder eyeshadow (8).
Creamy vanilla pencil eyeliner (9).

lips
Bright fuchsia lipstick crayon (10).

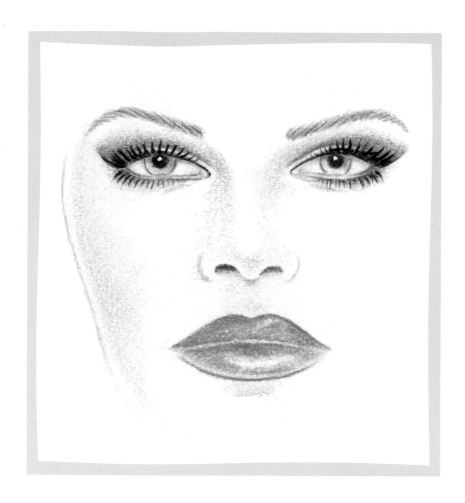

■ face

1 After prepping and priming Tamara's face (see pages 28–9), I used color correctors (see pages 30–1) to conceal any teenage blemishes and to add brightness underneath her eyes.

2 I wanted to keep the skin looking fresh, so I chose a tinted moisturizer for light coverage that would even out her skin tone without covering up her youthful radiance. Then I set it with a light dusting of translucent powder.

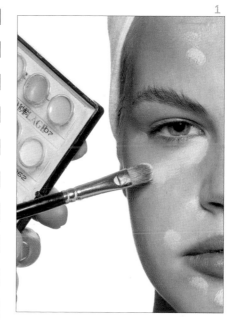

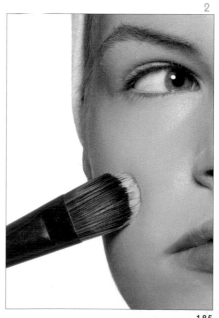

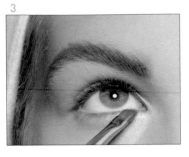
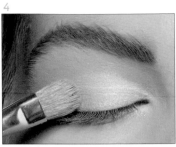
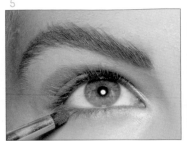
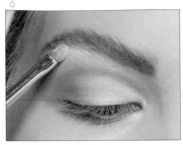

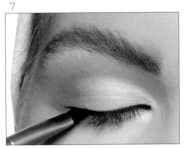
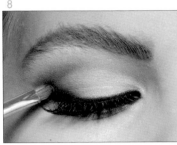
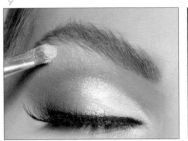
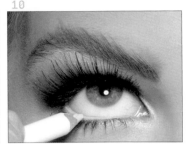

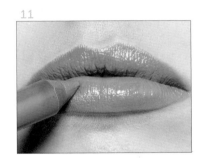

◼ eyes

3 As Tamara is blonde, she doesn't need to pluck her brows much, so I just tidied them up and kept them as natural as possible. After plucking away any stray hairs without exaggerating her gentle arch, I brushed her brows up and filled in any gaps with a light ash-blonde brow powder. Using a small angled brush, I applied a vanilla pigment to the inner corner of the eyes, taking it to the middle of the eyelid and lower lash line. Adding brightness to this area "lifts" the eyes and makes them look more alert. Make sure you use a warm tone that complements your skin tone—nothing too white or with a blue undertone, as this will look too stark.

4 Then, with a medium eye brush, I added a shimmery cotton-candy-pink eyeshadow to the outer half of the eyelid and blended the edges together to create a soft, dreamy pastel-pink eyelid.

5 Using a small pencil brush, I fed hot-pink powder eyeshadow into the socket line and onto the outer corner of eye. I then swept it from the outer corner under the lash line to meet the vanilla pigment, fading the colors together so they graduate from light at the inner corner to dark at the outer corner.

6 I applied a touch of vanilla pigment just below the brow bone and then blended the hot-pink in the socket line up to the brow bone. The shimmery pigment highlights the area and opens up the eye even more. Don't overdo this if you have heavy, hooded lids, as shimmery products on the brow bone will accentuate them; they can also be aging, as they will highlight any fine lines.

7 Next, I drew a fine line of black gel eyeliner as close to the upper lash line as possible. I also painted it lightly onto the base of her lashes, which are quite fair. This creates depth and gives maximum definition before applying mascara.

8 I curled her upper lashes, applied black mascara, and then added a feathery strip of false lashes for that real Barbie-doll look. I then added more eyeliner to create greater depth at the base of the lash line, lifting the liner at the outer corner to create a subtle flick, and layered black matte eyeshadow over this to soften the line. I blended a little of this eyeshadow into the outer corner of the eye, merging it with the hot-pink to create a soft purple that tones down the look and ensures it isn't too overpowering.

9 I added a little more vanilla pigment beneath the eyes at the inner corners and to the mid-section of the lid and under the brow bone. This gives a glossy, high-shimmer finish that really makes the eyes pop.

10 After adding another coat of mascara to the roots of the top lashes and to the bottom lashes, I applied a creamy vanilla pencil eyeliner to the bottom waterlines to open up and brighten the eyes.

◼ lips

11 I chose a bright fuchsia lipstick crayon for her lips. These crayons offer a quick and easy way to get color on the mouth without the need for a separate liner. You can get sheer ones, but I chose one with more coverage and applied two coats, blotting them in between applications, for a bold finish.

◼ finish

I chose a candy-pink blush to keep her face looking youthful, and blended it into the apples of the cheeks to bring out the natural contours. I then applied highlighter just above the cheeks to give the skin a little extra sheen.

think pink

Try different shades of pink to see what suits you. An old-fashioned tip for finding the perfect shade of pink lipstick is to smile and look at the color of your gums. Here are some ideas.

fair skin Go for petal pink (above), lilac pink, or peach pink.

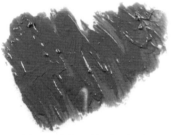

medium skin You're lucky, as most shades will suit you, but I'm more drawn to watermelon pink (above) and nude pinks.

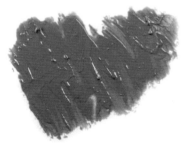

dark skin Try bright, bold pinks, magenta, purple-toned (above), and nude pinks.

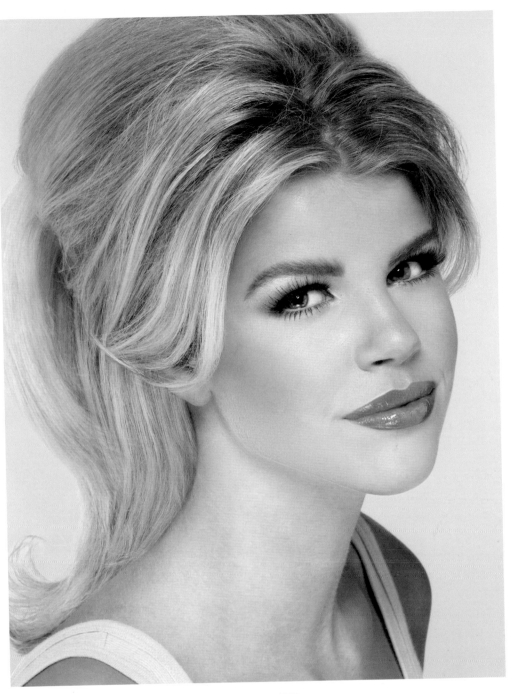

"I think every girl wants to feel pretty in pink and I absolutely loved the whole experience. I love pink but never knew how to make it look good on my face. I do now. #love, #make-up, #girlie, #pink, #beautiful."

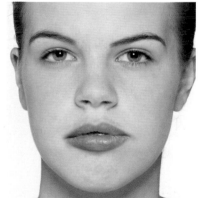

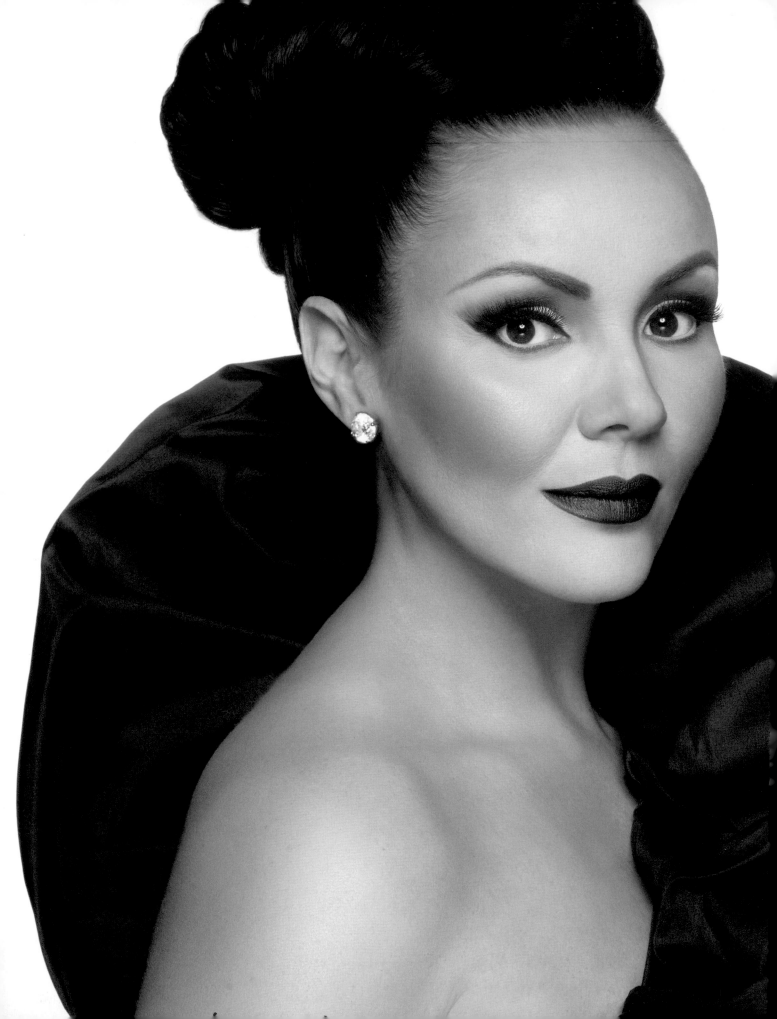

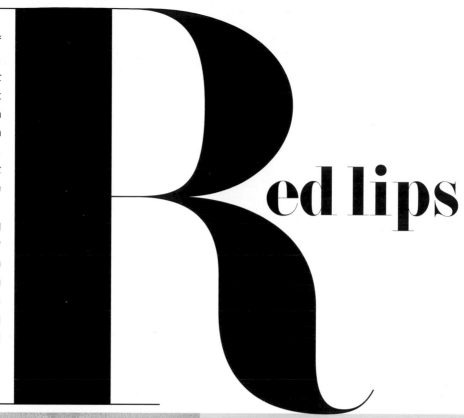

Red lips

The epitome of glamour and sexiness, red lipstick is never out of fashion—yet I've heard a million excuses from women for not trying it, whether it's their age, skin tone, the shape of their lips, or just not feeling brave enough to carry it off. But the truth is red lipstick can suit anyone; it's just about finding the right shade and texture for you.

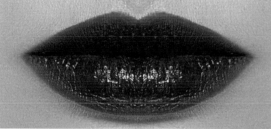

fair skin Shades of red with blue or pink undertones will usually suit you best and a soft rose-red is always flattering. Matte textures will give a more intense color than light-reflective satin fnishes.

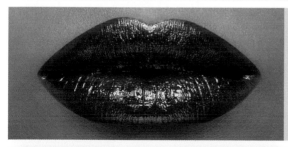

medium skin Yellow or orange-based reds in bright or deeper tones will usually suit those with medium skin tones. A rich cherry-red is a great choice. Try using two toning shades to contour the lips.

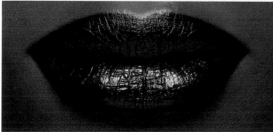

deep skin As a rule, the darker the skin tone, the deeper or brighter the color you can take. Anything from bold orange to brick-red, or from pinky reds with blue undertones to deep berry and burgundy.

Match the look and finish to the occasion—a sheer balm or a bee-stung stain strikes a very different note from a chic matte or a sexy gloss. The gorgeous actress Martine McCutcheon shows us how it's done (opposite). Her classic, velvety matte, scarlet lips are paired with glamorous eyes contoured in warm neutrals for a timeless red-carpet look that offsets her fabulous raven hair and fair complexion.

Perfect sexy lips

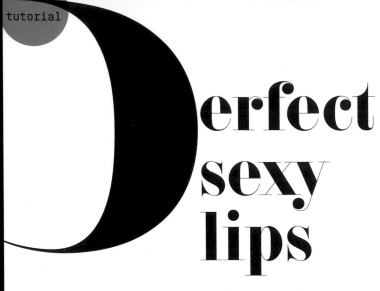

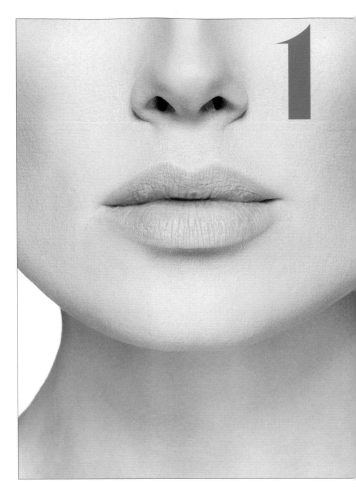

Contouring the lips by highlighting and shading is the way to achieve the ultimate 3-D pout. Whatever color you want to use, choose three complementary shades within the same tonal range—a creamy matte pencil in the darkest shade and lipsticks in a mid and lighter shade. Blue-based reds suit cool skin tones and orange-based reds work best on warm skin tones [see page 189].

1 For anything other than a sheer, barely-there look, start by neutralizing the natural pigment in the lips with lip primer or foundation. You can just use whatever is left on your brush or sponge after applying your base. This will keep the color of the lipstick true.

2 Brush translucent powder over the foundation to set it. A dry base will help your lipstick stay in place and last longer.

3 Apply highlighter just above the Cupid's bow with a small angled brush, following the shape of the lip. Use an illuminating cream or a light-reflecting powder two to three shades lighter than your skin tone. This emphasizes the Cupid's bow and is a good trick to make lips look fuller.

4 Using a contouring kit, or a cream or powder foundation two shades darker than your skin tone, apply a touch of shading just under the center of the lower lip. This pulls the lip forward, creating the perfect pout.

5 Starting at the center of the Cupid's bow, line the lips with a soft, creamy, matte pencil in the darkest shade. Make sure the point is sharp for absolute precision and take your time to make sure the outline is completely symmetrical. Using lip liner prevents lipstick from "bleeding."

6 Once the outline is complete, use small feathery strokes to bring the darkest color inward onto the outer quarters of the lips, leaving the middle clear.

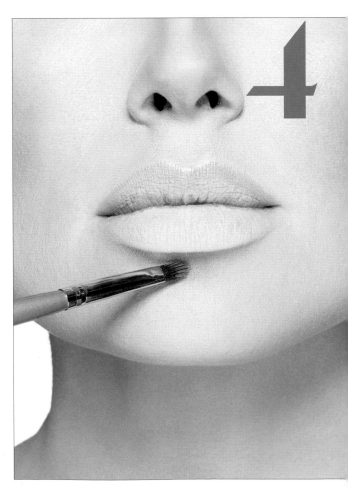

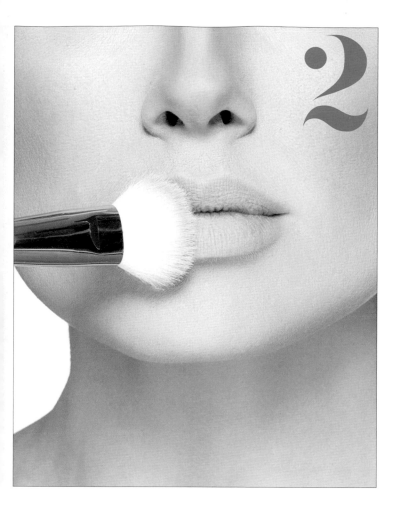

2

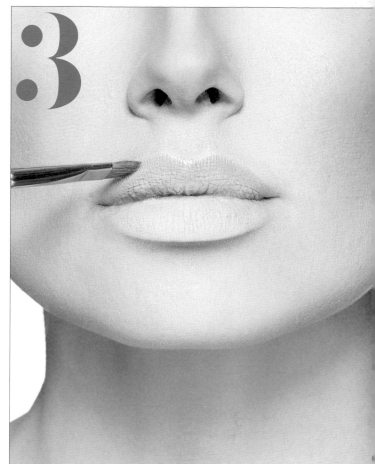

3

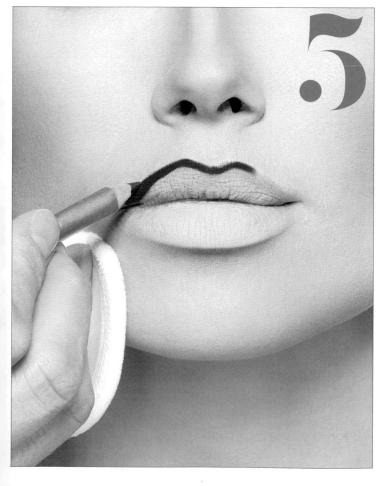

5

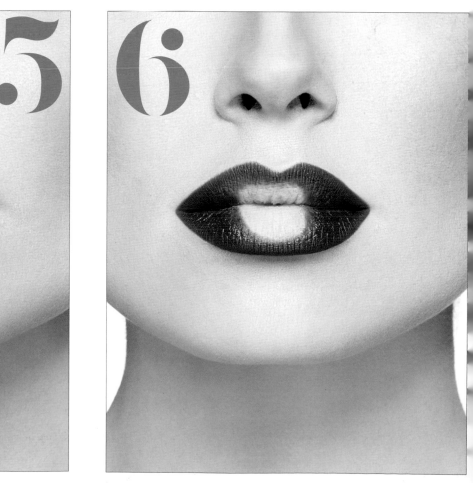

6

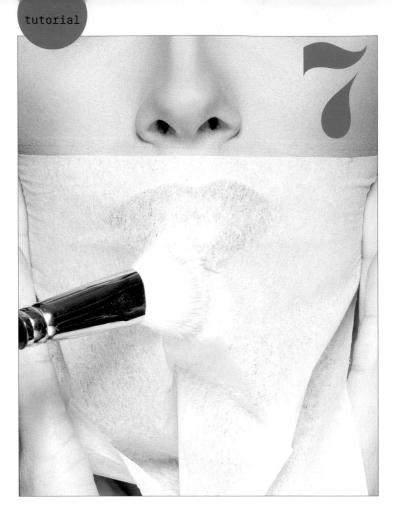

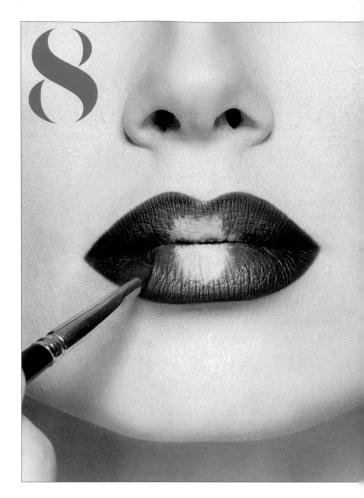

7 Blot with a tissue to get rid of any residue and set the color like a stain on the lips. With a little translucent powder on your brush, dab it over the tissue to absorb any moisture. Apply another layer of color with the pencil and blot again to intensify the depth of color.

8 Using a lip brush for precision, apply matte lipstick one shade lighter than the pencil to the next part of the lip, working inward and blending it over the pencil stain but still leaving the center of the lips clear. Blot the lips again and repeat to intensify the color and make the lipstick last longer.

9 Apply the lightest shade of lipstick to the center of the lips. Blot and repeat for a perfect matte or satin finish. If you wish, add a little gloss to the middle of the lower lip to enhance it even more—you can use a clear gloss or a gloss with pigment for even more of a pop.

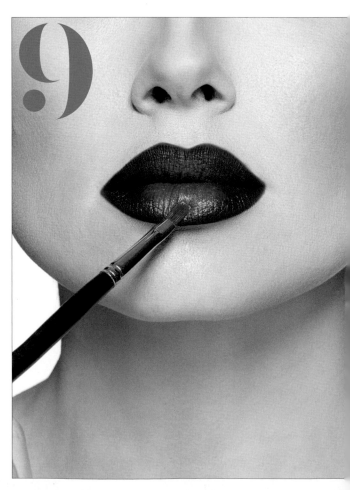

Remember:

To make a more pronounced pout, apply a darker tone around the outer edge of the mouth and keep the center lighter.

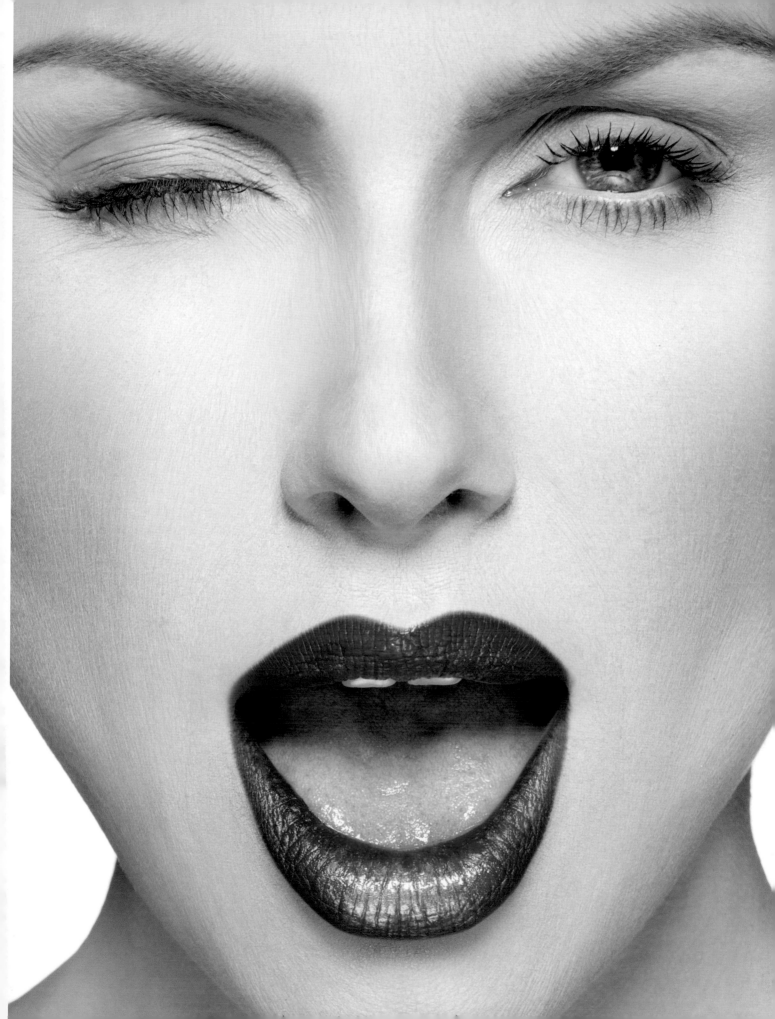

Bombshell

Nothing says "glamour" more than perfectly groomed, arched eyebrows framing the face, a sexy cat's-eye flick, and the reddest of red lips.

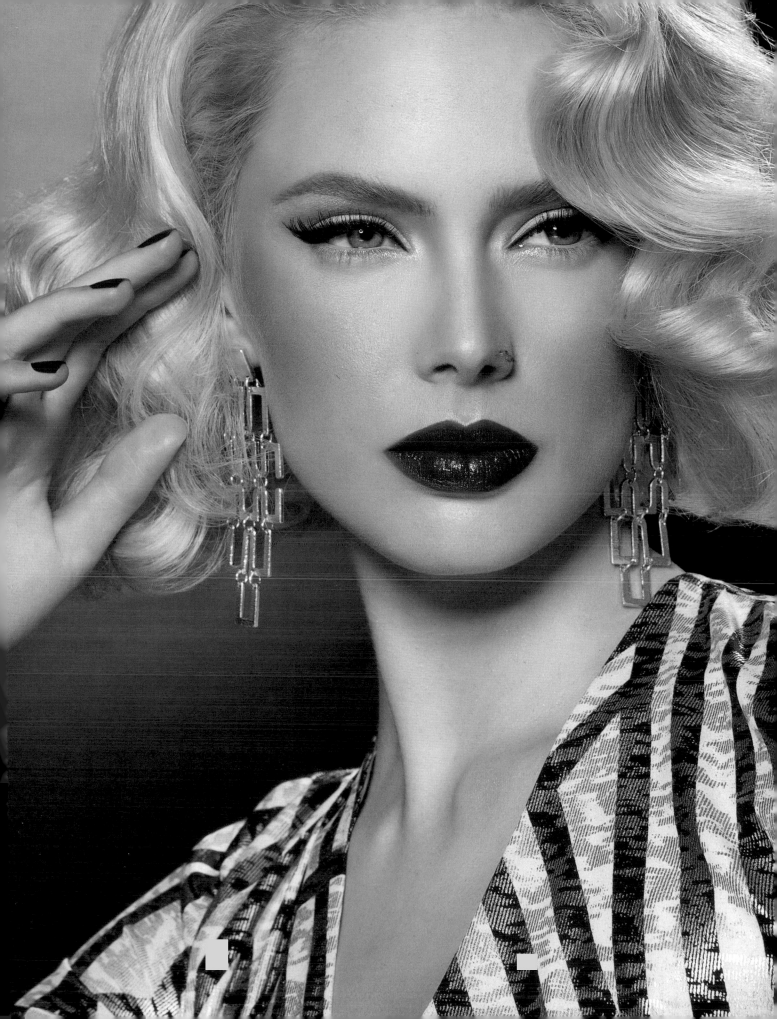

Bombshell Transformation

The seductive Bombshell look is epitomized for me by the Hollywood stars of the golden age, but it's not exclusive to blondes like Marilyn Monroe and Jayne Mansfield—think of redhead Rita Hayworth and brunette Jane Russell. The look is sexy but sophisticated, with a glamorous feline flick and fluttery false lashes that elongate the eyes and a creamy, flawless complexion that sets off the stop-sign-red, pillowy lips. The drop-dead gorgeous lips are the focus of this smoldering look and can be matte, satin, or gloss; equally, the face can either be camera-ready matte or have a slight sheen. Our model [previous spread] is a platinum blonde with fair skin, so I decided to channel old-school Hollywood, with a matte finish on the face, a fifties flick on the eyes, and sultry, glossy lips. For the transformation on Abi, I used a light, liquid foundation to keep a slight sheen on her skin but gave the lips a velvety matte finish for a longer-lasting result. It takes a grown-up kind of confidence to pull off this full red-carpet look, so make sure you have the perfect figure-enhancing dress and killer heels, and then complete the picture by painting your nails bright red and doing your hair in a Marcel wave or pin curls.

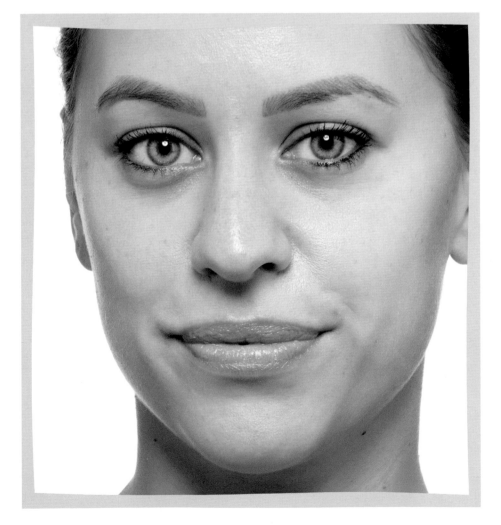

Abi is 28 and has the confidence and poise to wear this red-carpet look with flair. She has the perfect mouth for sexy red lips and I wanted to demonstrate how she could make her eyes look bigger and further apart by drawing in an exaggerated upward flick of eyeliner and a shadowy socket line for classic vintage cat's eyes.

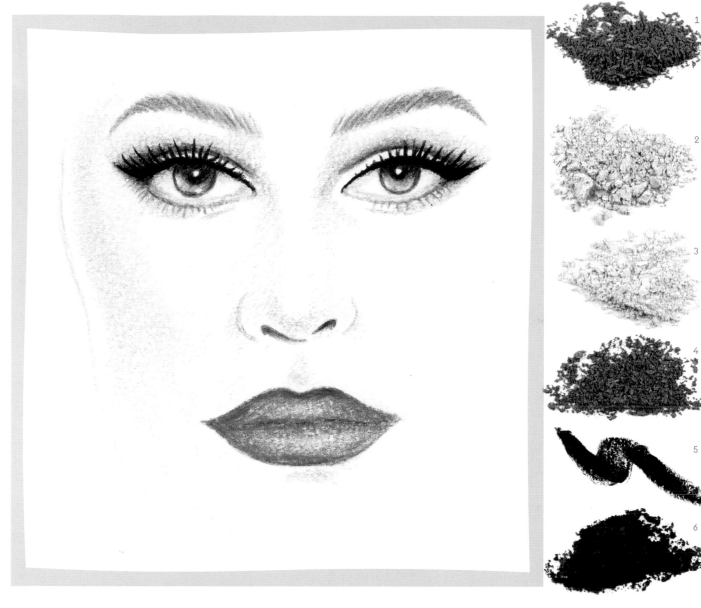

face

Cream foundation to match the skin tone and another two shades lighter for highlighting.
Translucent powder.
Dusky-brown matte powder for contouring.
Apricot-pink matte powder blush (1).
Champagne shimmer pigment (2).

eyes

Ash-blonde matte brow powder.
Ivory matte powder eyeshadow (3).
Mid-brown matte powder eyeshadow (4).
Black gel eyeliner (5).
Black matte powder eyeshadow (6).
Black mascara.
Full strip of fluttery false lashes that are longer toward the outer edge (7).

lips

Creamy scarlet lip pencil (8).
Matte, velvet-finish lipstick in the same rich shade (9).

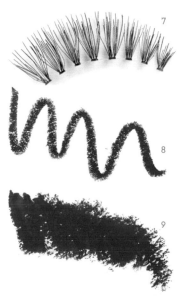

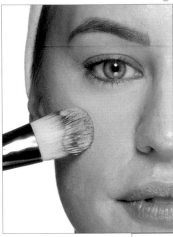

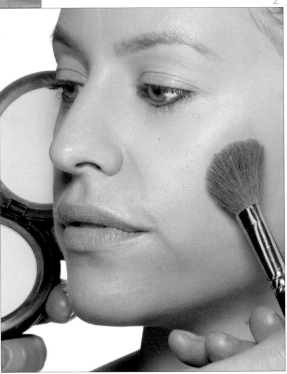

■ eyes

3 Having tweezed away any stray hairs, I emphasized her eyebrows with an ash-blonde brow powder, creating an elegant, strong arch. Abi's eyes are quite close-set, so my aim was to lift the arches of her brows and pull them outward. I did this by keeping the first half of the eyebrows soft and gradually deepening the color slightly from the peak of the arch as it slopes down to the outer tip. This draws more focus onto the outer part of the brows, which helps to "pull" the eyes apart.

4 For a neutral base, I applied ivory matte powder eyeshadow over the whole of the eyelid and up to the brow bone.

5 Next, I cut out a crease in a mid-brown matte powder eyeshadow, following the shape of her natural eye socket but taking it slightly higher, so the line is visible when her eyes are open. Emphasizing the socket gives the eyes depth and creates those heavy, Marilyn Monroe, "bedroom" eyes. When I was happy with the shape, I softly blended the edges into the ivory eyeshadow, so it's not a hard line.

6 Then I drew a feline flick along the upper lash line with black gel eyeliner and a small angled brush (see page 150). This is another great way to pull close-set eyes apart. The trick is to make the flick thicker toward the outer edge of the eye and pull it out and upward, but for this look I never connect the eyeliner with the socket line because I want to create as much space as possible on the eyelid. I went over the gel liner with black matte black eyeshadow to soften the line, give it more depth, and make it last longer.

7 I curled the upper lashes and applied a light coat of black mascara before adding a full strip of fluttery false lashes that get longer toward the outer edge to complement the feline flick.

8 I added more mascara to the base of the upper lashes, helping to create depth and blend Abi's natural lashes with the false set. A cat's-eye look is top heavy and the aim is to elongate the eyes as much as possible, so there is no make-up under the eyes, which would just make them look rounder again.

■ face

1 I prepped and primed Abi's skin as usual (see pages 28–9) and then lightly contoured her face with cream foundation. I chose one color that matched her skin tone and another two shades lighter to highlight any areas I felt needed brightening. I applied the matching foundation first and then added the lighter shade under her eyes, down the bridge of her nose and on its tip, on the center of her chin and forehead, and around the corners of her mouth. This is a softer approach to contouring and I blended the two tones well to create a radiant, flawless complexion.

2 I set the make-up with a light coat of translucent powder, taking care not to make her face too matte because I wanted the skin to retain a slight sheen. However, this look works equally well with a matte finish, so do whatever you prefer.

3

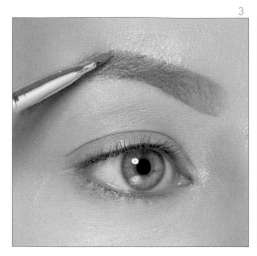

4

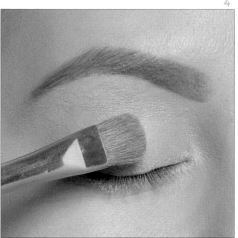

5

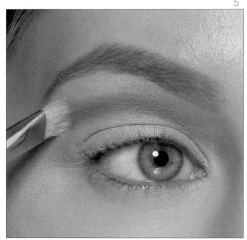

6

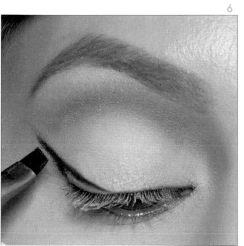

7

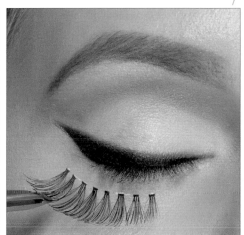

8

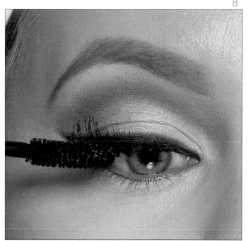

how to master a flick

» Take the eyeliner beyond
the end of the eye, angling it
upward; the longer the line,
the more dramatic it will be.

» Eyeliner is a personal thing,
so experiment to see what suits
you and decide how far you want
to push it.

» Practice getting the shape right
with a lighter-colored liner
and then go over it with the
black liner. Alternatively,
make dots where you want the
line to start and end.

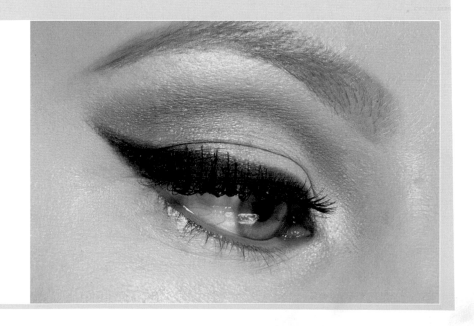

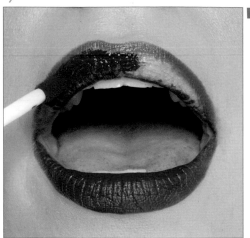

9

■lips

9 I finished the look with perfect, "old Hollywood" red lips. First, I created a symmetrical outline with a creamy scarlet lip pencil and then added a velvet-finish lipstick in the same rich shade. This high-pigment lipstick stains the lips and gives a velvety, matte finish.

■finish

Using a large angled brush, I lightly contoured and warmed up the cheeks with a dusky-brown matte powder and a soft apricot-pink matte blush. First, I emphasized the cheekbones and softened the temples with the brown powder, and applied blush to the cheeks, following the natural contour and taking it just as far as the apples. Then I highlighted the top of the cheekbones, around the beginning of the eyes, the tip of the nose, and the chin with a champagne shimmer pigment that brought her face to life.

how to master red lips

» Don't be scared of trying red lipstick because everyone can wear this color [see page 189].

» Always exfoliate your lips—flaky, dry skin is never a good look.

» Applying a lip primer or foundation first helps the lipstick stay in place. It also ensures the color of the lipstick will be true to the tube, as it won't be affected by your natural lip color.

» If you need to even out the shape of your lips, or make your mouth look smaller or larger, use concealer to block out your natural lip line [see pages 166-7].

» Apply a creamy lip liner around the edge of your lips to prevent the lipstick from "bleeding"—you can't do red lips without it.

» To create the perfect outline, line your lips with a nude pencil first and then go over it with your chosen red pencil.

» Blot each coat of pencil and lipstick with a tissue. This helps to prevent the color from smudging and makes it last longer.

» Brush translucent powder over your lips after you've applied the lipstick to absorb the oil and create a matte, stain-like finish that will last longer.

» Smear clear lip balm or petroleum jelly onto your front teeth to prevent your lipstick from sticking to them.

» Using two tones of lipstick—the slightly darker shade on the top lip and the lighter one on the bottom lip—makes the bottom lip look fuller.

» Glossy red lips will be more high-maintenance than matte ones, but if you want to add gloss, just put a dab on the middle of the bottom lip—don't put any on the top lip or you'll end up with a river of gloss that gets everywhere.

» When you've done your lips, pop your finger in your mouth and pull it out again. This gets rid of any excess lipstick on the inside of your mouth before it gets on your teeth.

» It's not the most ladylike of tips, but lick the rim of your glass before drinking, then your lipstick won't stick to it.

» For a daytime take on this look, just apply the eyeliner and mascara, and use a red stain on the lips.

» Complement this make-up with bright red nails and a glamorous Marcel wave.

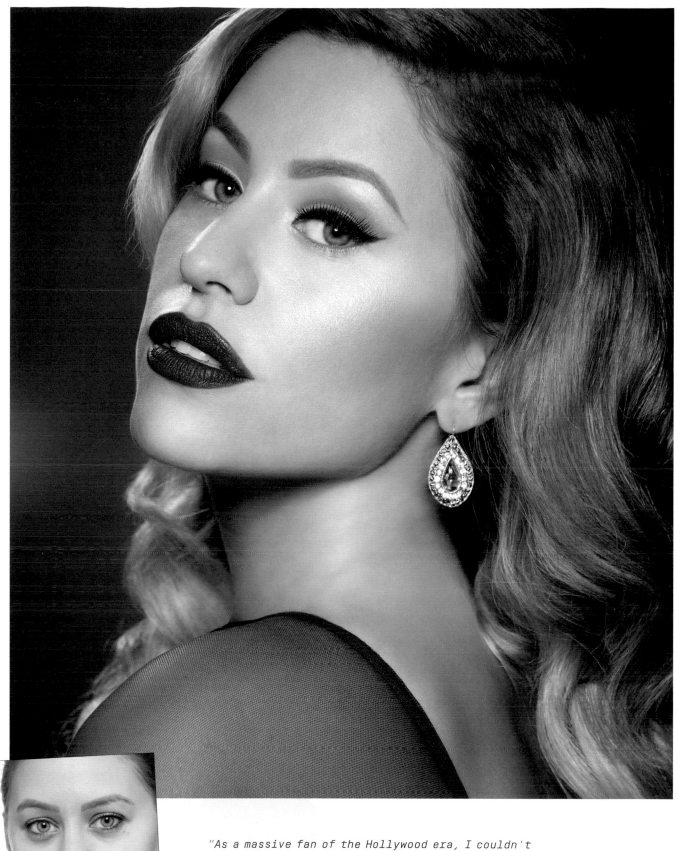

"As a massive fan of the Hollywood era, I couldn't wait to see what Gary was going to do. I don't usually wear red lips but the shade he used complemented my skin tone perfectly. It was so amazing to be turned into a fabulous screen siren and to realize I could actually do this at home."

Glamour puss

This is my take on the high-impact make-up of the late 1980s, with full brows framing strongly defined eyes and a bold, glossy mouth.

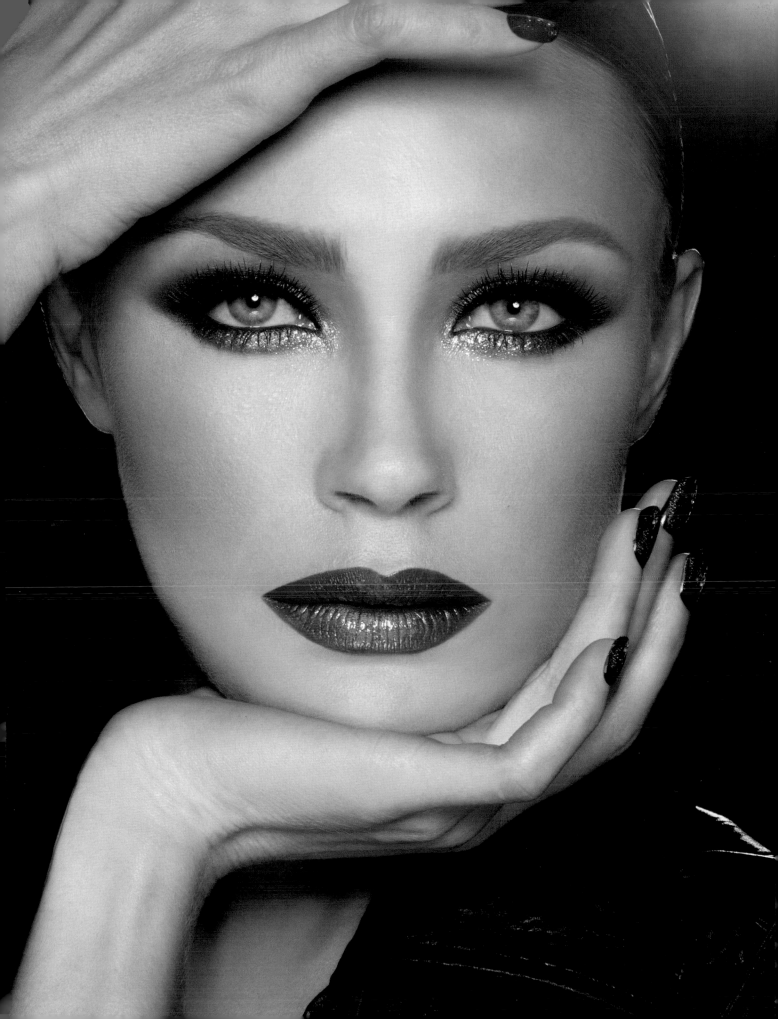

Glamour-Puss Transformation

Excess is the buzzword for this look, which places equal emphasis on the eyes and lips with neither taking center stage at the expense of the other. The rule that states you should play up only the eyes or the lips but never both at once is thrown aside, with the proviso that you need good eyes and a good mouth, as the make-up draws attention to both. The 1980s was about power dressing and a celebration of strong women, so make-up was bold, with eyes and lips defined for maximum impact. Divas of the decade were Joan Collins, Jerry Hall, Whitney Houston, and Madonna. The preferred palette included bold purples, blues, and greens, with all tones

of red, from scarlet to burgundy, on the lips. The guitar-playing models in Robert Palmer's "Addicted to Love" video were the inspiration for our model's make-up [previous spread]. The lips are a luscious claret shade with a mirror-like shine, and the heavily made-up eyes are dramatic, with emerald-green and sapphire-blue pigments and a touch of gold sparkle for a disco vibe. For the transformation on Charlie, I decided strong purple hues on the eyes and bold red lips would make the most of her blue eyes and full mouth. My challenge was to redraw her brows to frame the rest of the make-up. It's a face-changing process that blew her away.

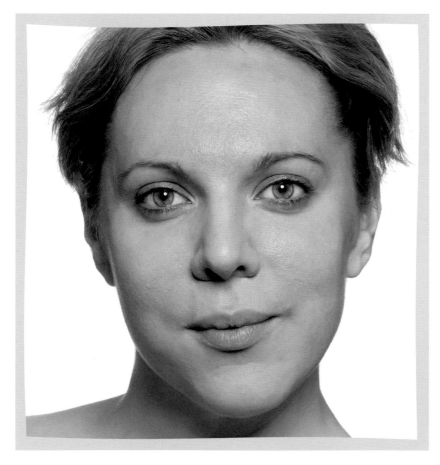

Charlie is 35 and loves experimenting with make-up and trying out different looks but admits she doesn't always get it right. She's got the personality to carry off this full-on look and relished the chance to feel like a glamour puss.

face
Mattifying primer.
Cream foundation to match
the skin tone.
Lighter and darker shades of cream
foundation for contouring.
Translucent powder.
Soft apricot powder blush (1).
Champagne-colored
highlighter (2).

eyes
Ash-blonde matte brow powder.
Bone-colored matte powder
eyeshadow (3).
Violet matte powder eyeshadow (4).
Purple matte powder eyeshadow (5).
Black gel eyeliner (6).
Black matte powder eyeshadow (7).
Black mascara.
Clusters of false lashes (8).

lips
Scarlet creamy lip pencil (9).
Scarlet satin or matte lipstick (10).
Clear lip gloss.

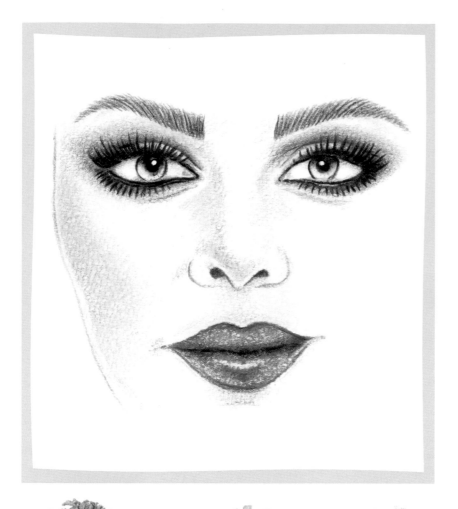

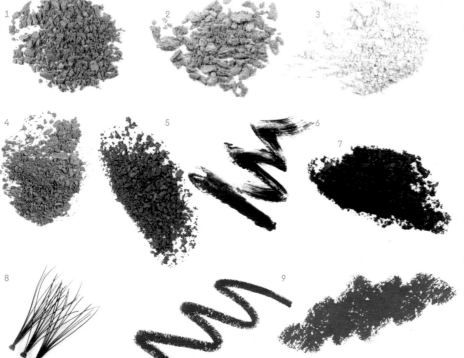

face

1 After prepping Charlie's face (see pages 28–9), I applied a mattifying primer followed by a light cream foundation all over the face to create a smooth base and an even skin tone. I then contoured her face with lighter and darker shades of cream foundation (see pages 56–61), concentrating on cutting out her cheekbones, slimming down her nose, and making her forehead look smaller.

2 I blended the edges well for a flawless finish and then set the make-up with translucent powder.

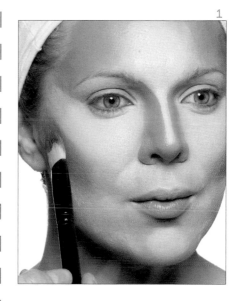

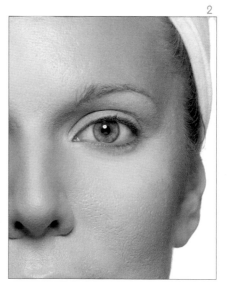

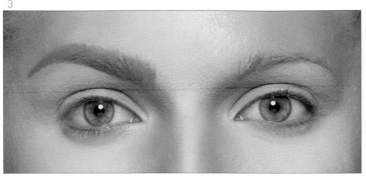
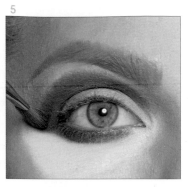
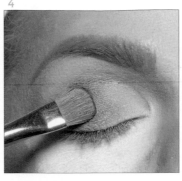

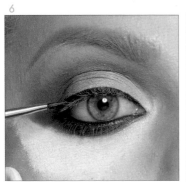
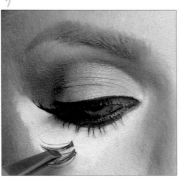
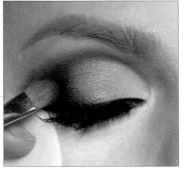
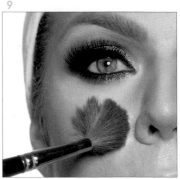

◼ eyes

3 First, I groomed her eyebrows, which were uneven and sparse in areas. She had overplucked her brows and removed hairs from the wrong places, resulting in an unflattering half-moon shape. She'd also plucked too much from the beginning of the brows, making the gap between them far too big, which makes her nose and forehead look larger. One of the key elements of this look is a full brow—wild but groomed. Choosing the correct product for filling in and drawing a new brow is really important. Some people like to use a pencil but I prefer a small angled brush and a matte powder or clay—any shine or shimmer will not look like a real brow. Getting the right tone is also key—here, I chose a brow powder with an ash-blonde tone because Charlie is fair. I redrew a new high arch, starting the brow a little nearer to the top of the nose to pull that area together and create better symmetry. This lifted her eyes and created the perfect frame for the rest of the make-up.

4 I applied a bone-colored matte powder eyeshadow over the whole eyelid to create a neutral base. Before I applied any colored eyeshadow, I brushed a light layer of translucent powder under the eyes to protect the skin from any fallout. Then I applied a violet matte powder eyeshadow to the outer half of the eyelid and blended it softly so that it fades into the bone-colored base toward the inner corner.

5 Next, I defined the socket crease with a purple matte powder eyeshadow using a pencil brush (matte eyeshadow gives a stronger effect than shimmer shadow, which diffuses the color and creates a softer finish). I blended this darker color into the outer corner and swept it under the lower lash line, making it darker and more dramatic at the outer corner and softening the intensity as I got closer to the tear duct. I then blended all the edges to create a dreamy effect.

6 For maximum impact, I applied black gel eyeliner to the top and bottom waterlines. I then added it to the upper lash line and blended black matte powder eyeshadow over it to create a softer, smudged effect. I also blended this into the purple eyeshadow under the lower lash line for more depth.

7 I curled her upper lashes and added a coat of black mascara to the top and bottom lashes. Then I added clusters of false lashes to fill out her upper lashes. Charlie has round, protruding eyes, so I used longer lashes at the outer corner of her eyes and shorter ones toward the beginning of her eyes to elongate them and pull them apart.

8 To increase the drama, I relined the upper lash line with the black gel liner and went over it again with the black matte eyeshadow. I then blended a little black eyeshadow onto the outer corner of the eyes and into the outer edge of the crease. I also smudged a little more under the lower lash line at the outer edge of the eye and blended it all well to give the purple more depth and graduation of tone.

9 Lastly, I added more black mascara to the roots of the upper lashes and to the bottom lashes. When the mascara was dry, I swept away the translucent powder from beneath her eyes with a soft brush.

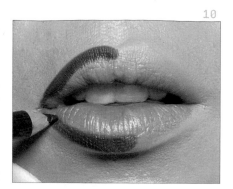

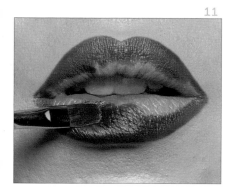

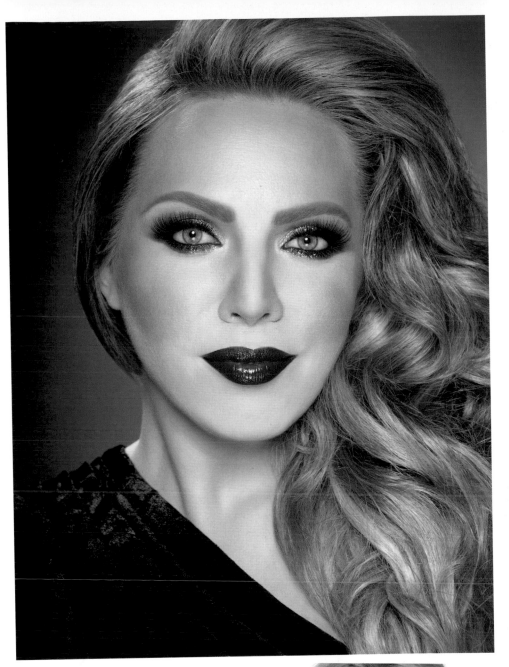

■lips

10 I wanted this to be the lips of all lips, so I chose a classic scarlet to flatter her skin (see page 189). First, I lined the lips using a creamy pencil, concentrating on creating a perfect, symmetrical shape.

11 When I was happy with the shape, I took the pencil onto the first half of the lips all the way round. I blotted this with a tissue and then applied the lipstick with a brush. I blotted the lips again, reapplied, and blotted again (see also pages 190–3). I finished the lips with a dab of gloss on the bottom lip and let it work its way around for a luscious pout.

■finish

For a healthy glow, I applied soft apricot powder blush, following the contour of her cheeks. I also added a touch of highlighter to the top of her cheekbones, the beginning of her eyes, and above her mouth to accentuate the fullness of her lips.

"I've never had my make-up done professionally so I jumped at the chance. I was absolutely blown away by the finished look. I started to cry, as I'd never seen myself look so beautiful. Gary literally changed my face— he's a phenomenon, a true artist, and an inspiration."

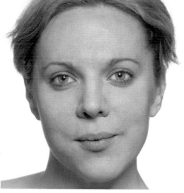

Tip For maximum drama, finish the look with sexy big hair or, for an edgier vibe, slick it back so that nothing steals the limelight from your power make-up.

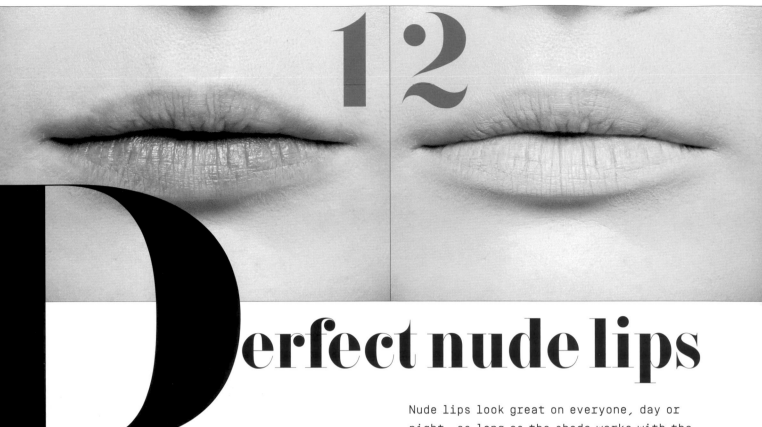

1 2

Perfect nude lips

Nude lips look great on everyone, day or night, as long as the shade works with the skin tone. Universally popular, they can be played down to look very understated or played up to look very sexy, and are the perfect complement to dramatic eyes.

1 Start by exfoliating the lips to ensure they are smooth. If the lips are dry, apply a coat of lip balm or moisturizer, let it absorb into the skin and then blot off any excess with a tissue.

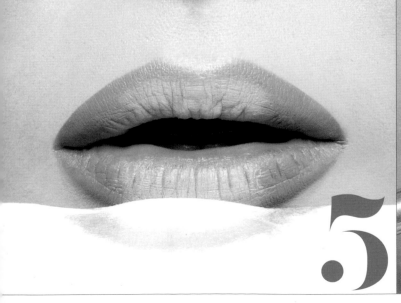

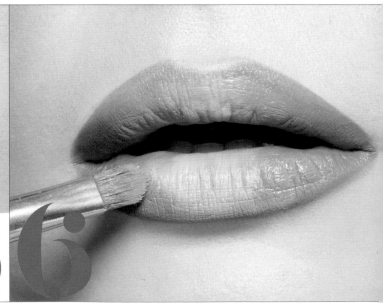

5 6

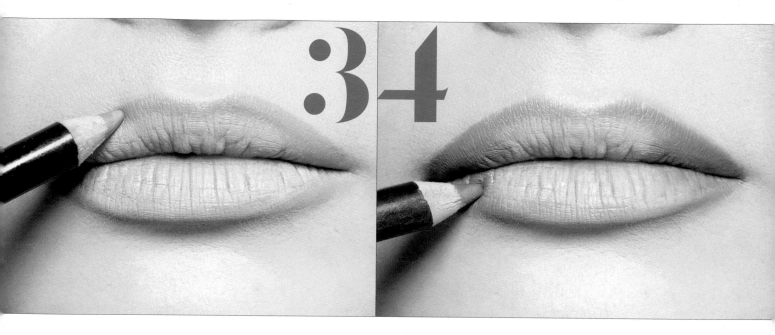

2 Apply lip primer, concealer, or foundation to the lips—you can just use what's left on your brush, as it must be the same as what's on your skin. This smooths the surface and neutralizes the natural lip color so it won't affect the color of the lipstick. It also helps hold the lipstick in place.

3 Pick a soft, creamy lip liner that glides on smoothly in a nude color that works with your skin tone. I usually choose one a shade darker than the lipstick to create a 3-D effect, but some people like to match it exactly. If you have great lips, simply outline the shape following the natural lip line; if you need to correct the shape, draw just inside or outside the lip line, depending on what you want to achieve (see pages 166–7).

4 Once you're happy with the outline, start to contour the lips by applying the lip liner to the outer edges of the mouth,

top and bottom, leaving the mid-sections free of color. The darker shade makes the edge of the mouth recede slightly, so that when you add the lighter color in the middle, it will make that area come forward and create a full pout.

5 Blot the lips with a tissue to fix the lip liner in place and create a stain on the lips. I sometimes repeat this two or three times, depending on how long I want the lipstick to hold.

6 Next, apply a creamy nude lipstick that complements your skin tone. Using a lip brush, apply the lipstick to the center of the lips, top and bottom, and then take it outward, merging it with the lip liner that is creating the illusion of depth.

7 Blot with a tissue to remove any excess oil.

8 Apply another coat of lipstick, as in step 6.

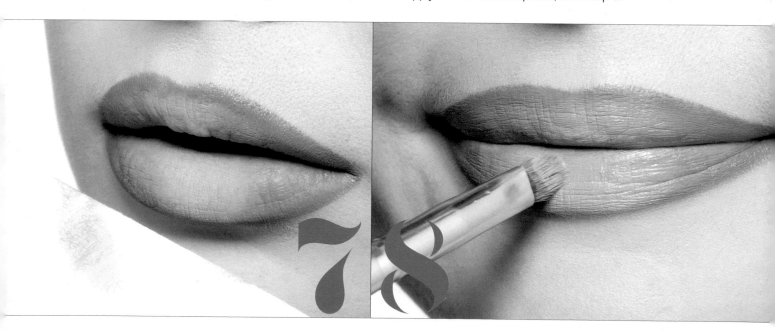

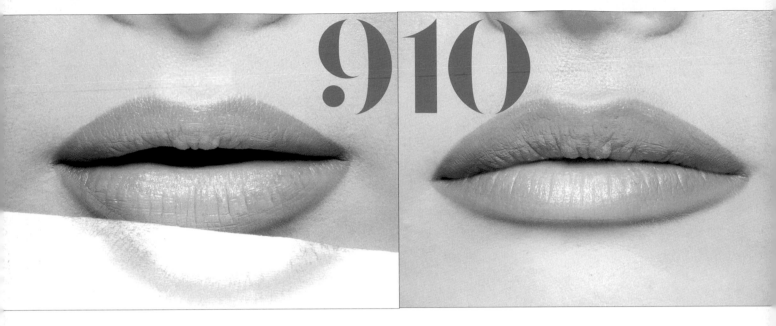

9 Blot the lips with a tissue again to create a stain on the lips and really build up the coverage, ensuring the lipstick will last longer without bleeding.

10 Depending on the effect you want to create, you can either leave the lips matte after blotting them or add a little bit of gloss. I wanted the center of the bottom lip to have a slight shine, to give it that sexy, Bardot-esque pout, so I added a dab of gloss. If you're using a satin lipstick, you could just apply a little more lipstick and not blot it.

11 With a small brush, add a touch of highlighter just above the top lip line, in the Cupid's bow, and around the top of the mouth. This accentuates the fullness of the lip and draws attention to the Cupid's bow.

12 Apply a touch of contouring cream or powder, one or two shades darker than your skin tone, under the bottom lip. This will make that area recede and the bottom lip look fuller.

nude shades to suit

fair skin Go for sheer, creamy, or satin nudes with pink or peach tones. Anything too beige will make you look pasty.

medium skin Look for nudes with orange undertones, such as shades of peach, beige, or caramel. Shimmering or metallic nudes or a touch of gold pigment look great with a tan.

dark skin Mocha and deep caramel tones look rich and luxurious, and clear, sheer nudes also work well.

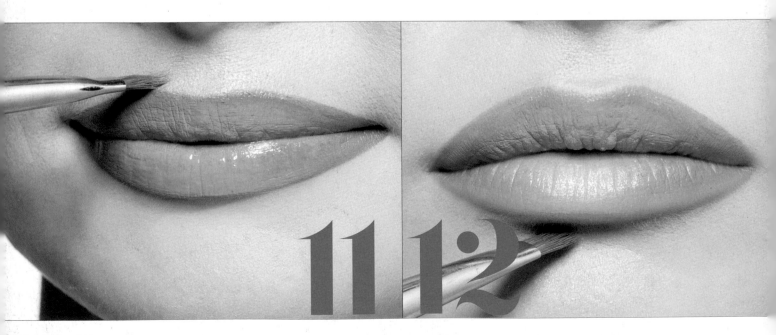

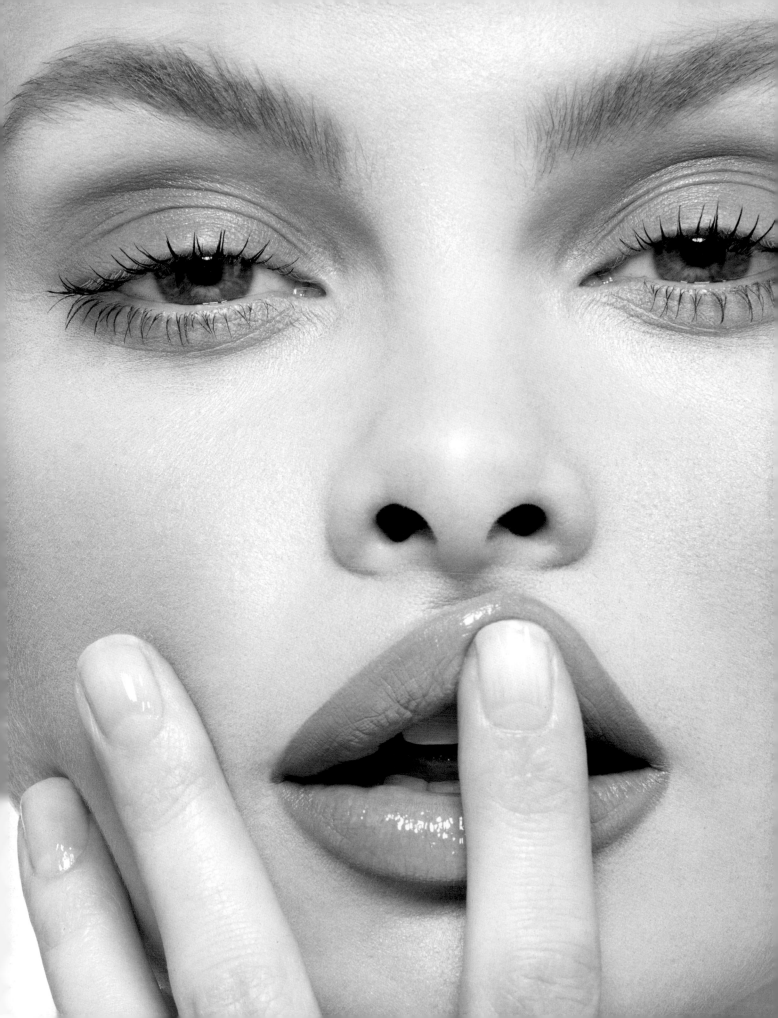

& Get up & go

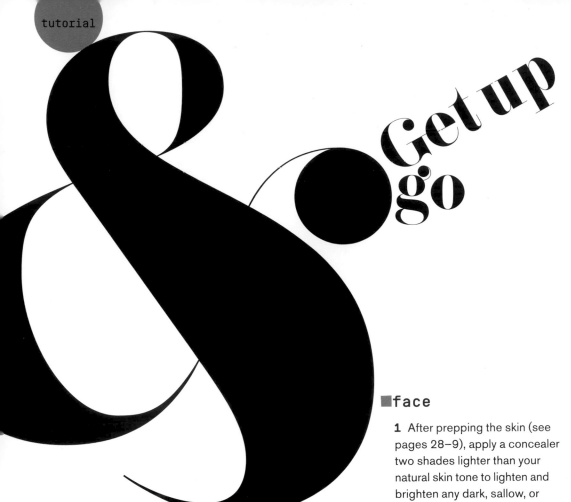
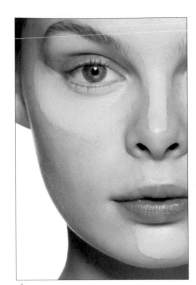

In our hectic lives, there are days when there isn't time—or, sometimes, the inclination—to apply a full face of make-up. But everyone still wants to make the best of themselves, and when time is not on your side, you need a make-up look you can create within minutes. Whether you're going shopping, to a meeting, or to lunch with a friend, this simple, low-maintenance make-up reflects an effortless freshness.

■ **face**

1 After prepping the skin (see pages 28–9), apply a concealer two shades lighter than your natural skin tone to lighten and brighten any dark, sallow, or red areas that need it, such as under the eyes, on the planes of the cheeks, on the bridge of the nose, under the corners of the mouth, and on the upper lip and chin. If you've got really good skin, this might be all you need and you can just blend it in and be good to go.

2 Most people need to apply a little light foundation all over the face to even out the skin tone. Apply a shade that matches your skin, using a sponge, a brush, or your finger, and merge it together with the concealer for a smooth, flawless finish.

3 Sweep a little translucent powder over the face to seal the foundation and eliminate any shine that usually occurs around the T-zone. As this is a fresh-faced look, don't overload the powder—keep it as natural as possible.

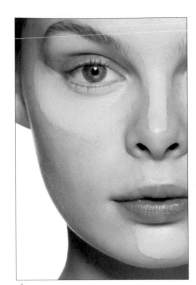

1

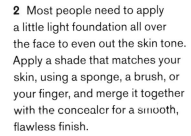

2

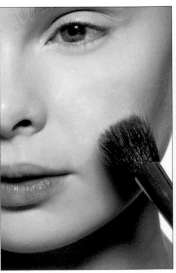

3

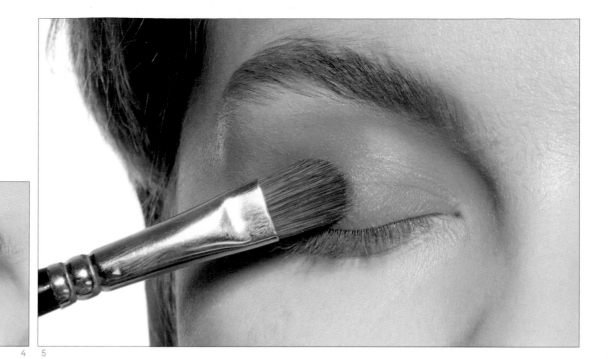

4   5

■eyes

4 Brush your brows into shape—this also removes any particles of powder that may have settled on the hairs. Keep your eyebrows looking very natural but fill in any gaps, if you need to, using a small angled brush and a little matte powder shadow or a brow pencil to create a shape you're happy with. If you're blessed with naturally great brows, you could just apply a touch of brow mascara to hold them in shape.

5 Choose a cream or powder eyeshadow with a slight shimmer or sheen in a soft, neutral shade that suits your skin tone. I always advise people to use warm tones for a no-make-up look, as cool tones can be too hard for a natural look. Sweep a wash of this color over your eyelids with a large flat eyeshadow brush and blend it into the skin well, especially at the outer edge of the eyes.

6 Change to a small round pencil brush and feed the same eyeshadow underneath the lower lash line from the outer corner, fading it toward the beginning of the eye. One tone over the whole lid is all you need to define the eyes and bring a bit of warmth to them.

7 Curl your lashes to open up your eyes and make them look bigger and more awake.

8 Add a soft sweep of black or dark brown mascara, depending on your coloring and preference. Apply it from the roots upward to create depth along the lash line and drag the wand out just before the ends to create a natural finish with no clogs or clumps.

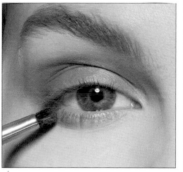

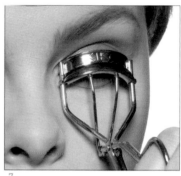

6   7

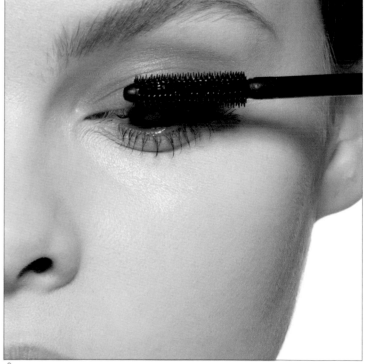

8

◼lips

9 Fill in your lips with a tinted lip gloss in a soft pink or peach shade that ties in with the eyeshadow you've used. For a more natural effect, you could use a colored balm—it all depends on how much color and pigment you want on the lips. If you would like to accentuate your lips slightly more, line them first with a creamy pencil in the same warm tone as the product you're putting on your lips.

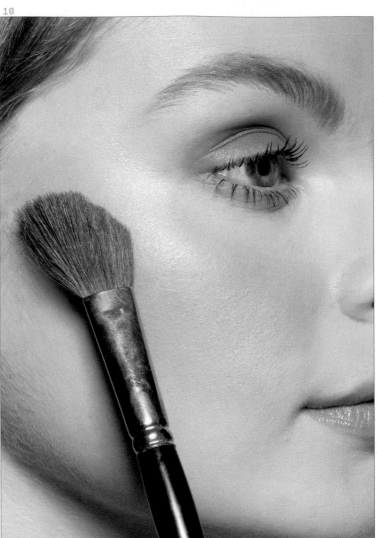

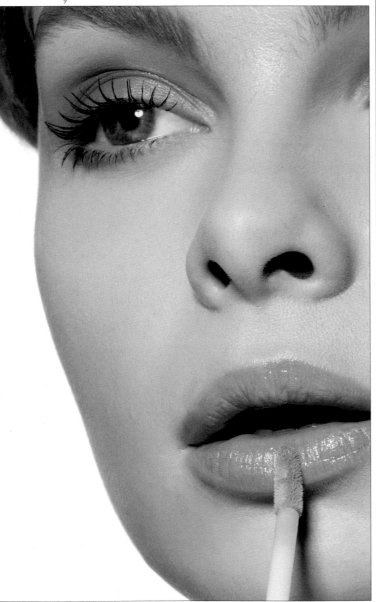

◼**10** Finally, apply a soft apricot powder blush along your cheekbones and onto the apples of the cheeks to create a natural flush that instantly warms up the face. Lightly sweep a little color onto your temples and under your jaw to carry the tone through.

Tip If you really have only minutes, do try a multipurpose product that you can use on your eyes, lips, and cheeks to give you a healthy, fresh look in no time.

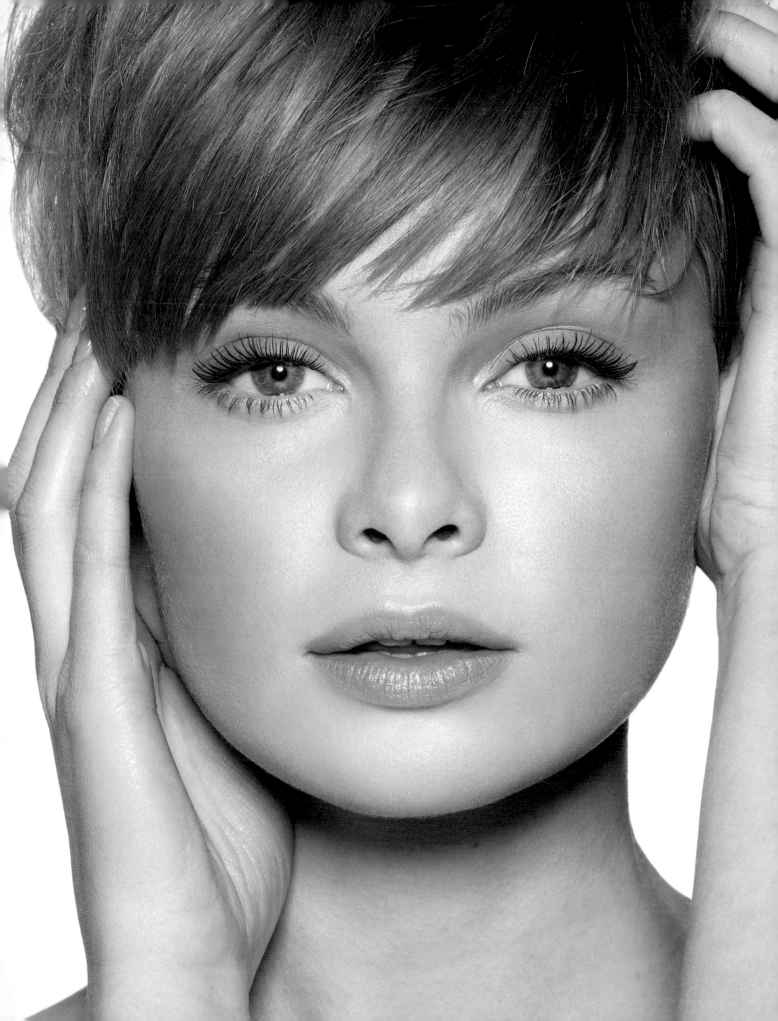

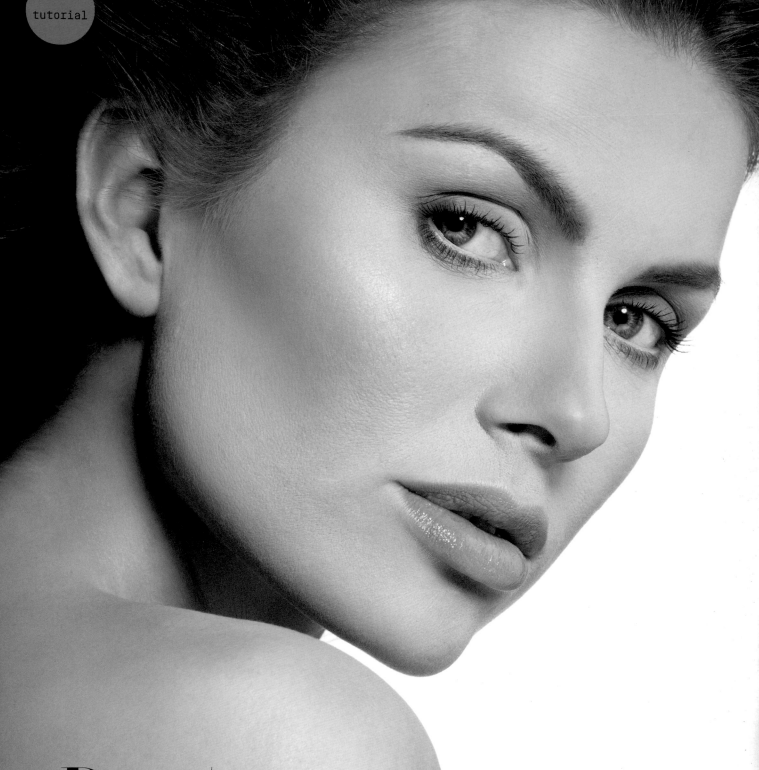

Day to Night

A natural, fresh daytime look can easily be glammed up for the evening with a few simple strokes of your make-up brush. For day, the emphasis is on fabulous skin, neat eyebrows, soft lips, and warm, complementary tones. For evening, keep to a similar color palette of rich caramel and honey tones, and add drama to the eyes with deeper shades, shimmery textures, and false lashes.

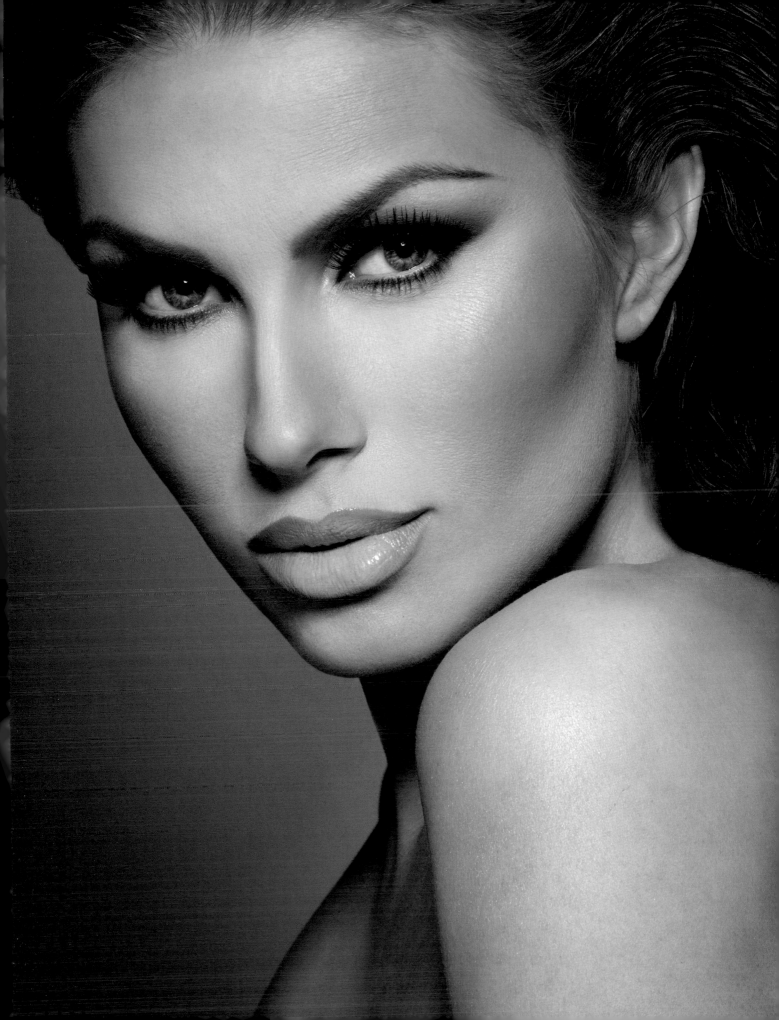

Natural daytime beauty

eyebrows Using a small angled brush, define the brows and fill in any gaps with brow powder or matte powder eyeshadow. If your natural brows are dark, choose a color one shade lighter; if your brows are very fair, go one shade darker. Add a touch of highlighter just underneath the brow bones to lift the brows and make the eyes look more awake.

cheeks If you are short of time, use a matte contouring powder to sculpt the cheekbones, sharpen the jawline, and warm up the temples; otherwise, lightly contour the face using light and dark shades of cream foundation (see pages 56–61). Apply a warm-toned highlighter to areas you want to brighten and an apricot cream or powder blush to the cheeks, then blend well.

skin Perfect skin is everything, so moisturize and prime (see pages 28–9), then apply a light foundation or concealer on the areas that need it, to even out the skin tone and cover any imperfections. A dewy finish looks fresh and youthful if your skin is naturally flawless, but a matte finish is more forgiving of any imperfections.

lips Apply a moisturizing nude, soft pink or peach balm or lipstick that matches your skin tone. A sheer, satin, cream, or matte finish all look good in the daytime, with a dab of gloss if you like. You can also add a touch of highlighter just above the upper lip to make it look fuller.

eyes Apply a wash of warm vanilla or nude eyeshadow to the lids—it can be matte or have a slight shimmer. Intensify the socket line with a complementary apricot or taupe shade, and blend well. For more definition, line the upper lash line with black matte powder eyeshadow using an angled brush. Curl the lashes and apply dark brown or black mascara.

Tip To awaken and brighten tired eyes, use a nude [off-white or ivory, not stark white] eyeliner pencil on the lower waterlines.

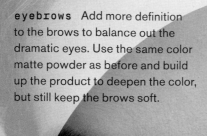

eyebrows Add more definition to the brows to balance out the dramatic eyes. Use the same color matte powder as before and build up the product to deepen the color, but still keep the brows soft.

skin and cheeks Touch up the contouring, if you need to, using the same products as before. Add light-reflecting highlighter to give the skin a radiant glow. Apply another layer of apricot blush and blend well. Set with translucent powder.

eyes
Work with three complementary eyeshadows: pale vanilla or nude, mid-apricot or warm brown (this can have a shimmer, if you wish), and dark brown. Brush the pale color under the brow bone and over the lid. Apply the apricot tone to the middle section of the lid and the dark brown to the outer corner. Blend the dark brown into the socket line, then bring it just under the lower lash line, softening it toward the inner corner—keeping the dark shade to the outer corner and socket line makes the eyes look further apart and bigger. Blend well so there are no hard lines.

lashes Using an angled brush, draw a thin line of brown or black gel liner along the roots of your upper lashes. Measure the false lashes against your lash line and trim off the outer edge to fit if you need to. Apply the glue, wait until it is tacky, then position the strip as close to the roots as you can, starting in the center and working out. When the lashes are stuck but before you open your eye, push them up from underneath for a natural curve. Seal the lash line with gel liner and apply mascara to the roots to blend the natural and false lashes together.

lips Prime your lips with foundation and powder to knock out their natural color and create a long-lasting base. Line the lips with a soft beige pencil, bring the color inward from the edge and blot, then fill in the lips with creamy nude lipstick. Blot and repeat. Keep the lips matte or satin, or add a dab of gloss to the lower lip.

shoulders and décolletage
Don't forget to contour and highlight your shoulders and décolletage if they are going to be on show.

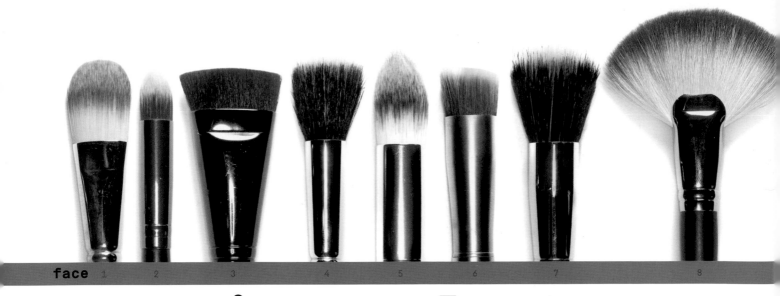

face   1   2   3   4   5   6   7   8

Favorite products

There are so many cosmetics brands offering great make-up and skincare products—with new colors and formulations being launched every month—that we are really spoilt for choice. Below are some of my favorites, but this is by no means an exhaustive list.

skincare

Alpha-H Liquid Gold. **Caudalíe** Beauty Elixir. **Charlotte Tilbury** Charlotte's Magic Cream. **Cult 51** Night Cream; Immediate Effect Serum. **Dr Paw Paw** Original Balm. **Emma Hardie** Moringa Cleansing Balm. **GLAMGLOW** Youthmud Tinglexfoliate Treatment. **James Read** Day Tan SPF 15 Face. **Kate Shapland** Legology Air-Lite Daily Lift for Legs. **Sarah Chapman** Skinesis Overnight Facial. **Sunday Riley** Good Genes Treatment, Serum & Mask. **Zelens** Z-22 Absolute Face Oil.

make-up

FACE **Amazing Cosmetics** Amazing Concealer. **Anastasia Beverly Hills** Pro Series Contour Kit. **bareMinerals** Mineral Veil Powder. **Ben Nye** Banana Luxury Powder; Rose Petal Luxury Powder; MediaPRO HD 18-Color Sheer Foundation Palette – Global. **The Body Shop** Honey Bronze Bronzing Powder; Vitamin E Cool BB Cream; Honey Bronze Face Gel. **Bourjois** Healthy Mix Foundation. **CHANEL** Perfection Lumière Long-Wear Flawless Fluid Makeup. **Charlotte Tilbury** Filmstar Bronze & Glow. **Crown Brush** 26 Shade Professional Contouring Palette. **Estée Lauder** Bronze Goddess Powder Bronzer. **Giorgio Armani** Luminous Silk Foundation. **Illamasqua** Skin Base Foundation; Satin Primer; Matte Primer; Gel Sculpt; Cream Blusher. **Kryolan** Perfect Matt Primer; Professional Blusher Set 15 Colours. **Laura Mercier** Secret Camouflage Concealer. **MAC** Studio Fix Powder Plus Foundation; Studio Sculpt SPF 15 Foundation; Studio Face and Body Foundation; Studio Fix Fluid SPF 15; Pro Conceal and Correct Palette; Prep + Prime Transparent Finishing Powder/Pressed; Powder Blush. **Make Up For Ever** HD Foundation. **NARS** Radiant Creamy Concealer; Body Glow. **Screenface** Dermacolor Palette K 24 Colours; **Sleek MakeUP** Face Contour Kit. **Smashbox** Photo Finish Foundation Primer. **Stila** Convertible Color Dual Lip and Cheek Cream. **Studio 10** Age Defy Skin Perfector; Youth Lift Glow-Plexion; Visible Lift Face Definer. **Tom Ford** Traceless Perfecting Foundation SPF 15. **Topshop** Cream Blush; Highlighter, Sunbeam. **Urban Decay** Naked Skin Weightless Ultra Definition Liquid Makeup. **BROWS** **Anastasia**

Beverly Hills DipBrow Pomade; Large Synthetic Duo Brow Brush. **Kiko** Eyebrow Marker. **EYES** **Barry M** Dazzle Dust; Super Soft Eye Crayon; Kohl Pencil; Eyeshadow Pencil. **Bobbi Brown** Long-Wear Cream Shadow; Long-Wear Gel Eyeliner. **Bourjois** Little Round Pot Intense Eyeshadow; Volume Glamour Ultra Black Mascara. **CHANEL** Illusion D'Ombre Long Wear Luminous Eyeshadow. **Charlotte Tilbury** Colour Chameleon; Luxury Palette Colour-Coded Eyeshadows. **Crown Brush** 28 Nude Eyeshadow Palette. **Illamasqua** Liquid Metal; Liquid Metal Palette; Pure Pigment. **Inglot** AMC Pure Pigment Eye Shadow. **Kryolan** Eye Shadow Primer; Glamour Sparks Eyeshadow. **Lancôme** Grandiôse Mascara. **MAC** Fluidline Gel Liner. **Make Up For Ever** Smoky Lash Mascara. **NARS** Duo Eyeshadow. **Studio 10** I-Lift Longwear Liner. **Tom Ford** Eye Defining Pencil; Extreme Mascara. **Urban Decay** Naked Eyeshadow Palettes 1, 2 and 3; Moondust Eyeshadow; Eyeshadow Primer Potion; Heavy Metal Glitter Eyeliner; 24/7 Glide-on Eye Pencil; Supercurl Curling Mascara. **Yves Saint Laurent** Volume Effet Faux Cils Shocking Mascara. **FALSE LASHES** **Ardell** Lashes. **DUO** Eyelash Adhesive White Clear. **Eylure** Lashes. **Gary Cockerill** Pro Lashes. **Kiss** Lashes. **Kryolan** Lash Adhesive Pro. **LIPS** **The Body Shop** Honey Bronze Shimmering Lip Balm. **Bourjois** Effect 3D Lipgloss. **CHANEL** Lèvres Scintillantes Glossimer; Le Crayon Lèvres Precision Lip Definer. **Clarins** Instant Light Lip Balm Perfector. **Joan Collins Timeless Beauty** Divine Lips Lipstick. **Make Up For Ever** Rouge Artist Intense Lipstick. **NARS** Velvet Lip Liner; Velvet Matte Lip Pencil. **Sleek MakeUP** Twist Up Lip Liner. **Stila** Sparkle Luxe Gloss; Magnificent Metals Lip Gloss. **Studio 10** Longlast Velvet Liquid-Lips; Age Reverse Perfecting Lipliner. **Tom Ford** Lip Color Shine. **Yves Saint Laurent** Rouge Pur Couture Lipstick; Volupté Sheer Candy Lipstick.

tools

Crown Brush Large Duo Fibre Face Brush; Deluxe Crease Brush; Jumbo Powder Blush; Deluxe Oval Foundation. **MAC** Brush Cleanser. **Real Techniques** Blush Brush; Deluxe Crease Brush; Buffing Brush; Stippling Brush. **Shu Uemura** Eyelash Curlers. **Tweezerman** Tweezers. **HAIR** **Annabel's Wigs** Hairpieces and Wigs. **Easilocks** Hair Extensions and Hairpieces. **Hair Rehab** Clip-in Extensions. **Hot Hair** Hairpieces. **Living Proof** Prime Style Extender Spray. **Peaches & Cream** Hairpieces. **T3** Bodywaver Professional Curling Iron. **Stephanie Pollard** Bespoke Hair Extensions.

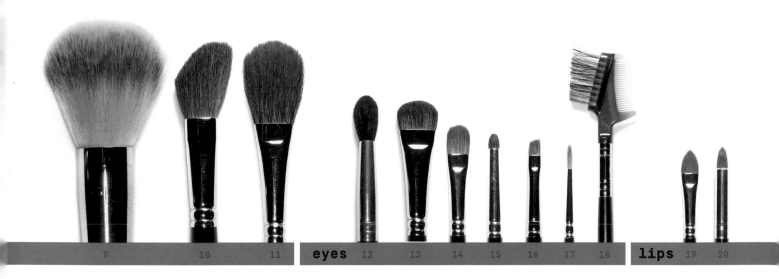

9   10   11   **eyes** 12   13   14   15   16   17   18   **lips** 19   20

essential brushes

Make-up brushes come in a variety of shapes, sizes, and textures for the face, eyes, and lips. The bristles are either natural—squirrel, pony, sable, kolinsky, or badger hair—or synthetic—nylon or polyester. Natural-fiber brushes vary in stiffness but tend to be fluffier and are best used for applying powder formulations. As a rule, the longer the fibers, the softer the brush will be. Smoother synthetic bristles are best for applying creams and liquids. Brushes are your most important make-up tool, so it's worth investing in good-quality ones that will last a long time if you look after them. A bad workman blames his tools, but you should get good results if you use the right brushes for the job. Here are some of my favorites (see above).

CLASSIC FOUNDATION BRUSHES (1, 2, and 5) come in different sizes and mostly have either a tapered or rounded shape. The bristles are synthetic, so they hold the fluid or cream well, spread it evenly over the face for a flawless finish, and are easy to clean. You can use them wet to create a lighter consistency. Use a large size (1) to apply foundation to the whole face, and a smaller brush with a tapered tip for adding detail or applying the product to awkward areas, such as around the eyes, hairline, and nose; the smallest brush (2) is ideal for applying concealer. You can also apply foundation with a wedge-shaped sponge, an egg-shaped beauty blender, or your fingertips.

CONTOURING BRUSHES are designed for sculpting the face by cutting out the cheekbones, defining the jaw, softening the temples, and slimming down or shortening the nose. They come with either synthetic or natural-fiber bristles for use with liquid, cream, or powder contouring products (3 and 6 are just two examples). Choose a size and shape suitable for the area of the face you are working on.

STIPPLING BRUSHES (4 and 7) are circular, flat-topped, two-tone brushes made up of a combination of natural and synthetic fibers. They can be used to apply all types of foundation by gently stippling, or tapping, the product into the skin and then buffing in a circular motion to create an airbrushed finish with no streaks.

FAN BRUSHES are used for powder products. They give a light touch and create very light coverage on the face. A large fan brush (8) is great for dusting the face with translucent powder, while smaller ones can be used for sweeping away fallout from under the eyes or applying highlighter to the top of the cheekbones.

CLASSIC POWDER BRUSHES have soft, natural-fiber bristles. A rounded/domed powder brush (9) is for buffing in a circular motion, while tapered or chiseled powder brushes are for dusting and sweeping powder onto the face. Always tap off the excess product from the brush before applying it to the face.

BLUSH/BRONZER/HIGHLIGHTING BRUSHES (10 and 11) are smaller than powder brushes and so give greater precision. They may be angled, rounded, or paddle-shaped, and the bristles are usually tightly packed at the base and softer at the tip for a natural finish.

EYESHADOW BLENDING BRUSHES (12) are soft and flexible with densely packed bristles and a soft, rounded tip, designed to fit into the crease of the eye. They are used to blend colors together and create a soft finish with no hard lines, and can also be used to apply eyeshadow.

FLAT EYESHADOW BRUSHES are for applying eyeshadow to the lid area. Everyone's eyes are different, so choose one to suit the size of your eyelid. The large, flat, natural-bristle brush (13) is designed to put as much product as possible on a large lid, giving a smooth, even coverage, while the smaller one (14) is ideal for smaller eyelids or for adding detail to an area of the lid.

PENCIL BRUSHES are small, compact brushes with either a flat or rounded tip (15). They are great for adding detail and you can use them to apply eyeshadow underneath the eye, in the crease, along the lash line, and on the beginning of the eye. You can also use them for blending.

SMALL ANGLED BRUSHES (16) come in a variety of sizes and are great multipurpose brushes that can be used with powder, cream, or gel eyeliner. They offer great precision for drawing in eyebrow shapes, cutting out creases, and defining waterlines and lash lines.

FINE EYELINER BRUSHES (17) are used for filling in lash lines and creating detail. They are best for applying gel or cream eyeliner, but you need a steady hand to create a perfect fine line.

A DUAL-PURPOSE BROW BRUSH AND LASH COMB (18) has a brush on one side for grooming the eyebrows and brushing them into shape, and a comb on the other side for separating eyelashes and removing clumps of mascara.

LIP BRUSHES (19 and 20) generally have synthetic bristles and come in different sizes to suit different lips. A large, flat brush (19) can be used for applying product to the planes of the lips, while a smaller tapered brush (20) gives more precision.

ndex

Figures in italics refer to captions and entries in italics refer to transformations.

acknowledgments

A very big thank you to everyone who made this book possible.

Huge thanks to Jacqui Small for listening to my ideas, enabling me to commit my vision onto paper, and for making the book happen, and to Grace Fodor, Founder of Studio 10 Makeup, for her help in getting the project off the ground and her support, guidance, and input throughout.

To the team who put the book together, helped shape the content, and made it so beautiful, thank you for your expertise and contribution. Especially my editor, Zia Mattocks, for making sense of my thoughts and putting them all down on paper so clearly and beautifully, and Lawrence Morton, for his artistic vision, talent, and fabulous design. You have both taken so much time and care to help me ensure the book is the best it can be and I have really valued your input as the project has evolved. A big thank you also to Vikki and Karl Grant for the stunning photographs and for their professionalism, flair, and commitment throughout those long days in the studio.

The book wouldn't have been possible without all of the wonderful people featured on its pages. A huge thank you to all the gorgeous women who let me transform them: Lynne Beavers, Ann Cockerill, Charlotte Coultard, Maica Garcia, Tamara Hindley, Hari Kamaluddin, Chloe Koy, Georgina Leavey, Mary McGovern, Leena Oh, Abbi Rose, Elle Paige Scrivins, and Charlie Wilkinson; and the stunning professional models: Andrea Ita at Hughes, Amy at MOT, Amy F at Nevs, Elly at MOT, Illy at Body, Laura R at MOT, Maisie at Profile, Michaela Ireland, Olga P at Profile, and Stacey H at Profile.

Very special thanks to the beautiful Kelly Brook, Chloe Green, Martine McCutcheon, Melanie Sykes, and Jo Wood, for their friendship and for giving up their time to take part in my book—your involvement is greatly appreciated.

Thank you to my wonderful friends Nick Gold, Laura Zilli, and Michael Evans, for all their help and support.

A big thank you to all the companies that so generously supplied products for the photoshoot, many of which are mentioned on page 220, especially Charles Fox, Screenface, and Kryolan.

Thanks also to Danny Buttleman at Shoreditch Studios.

And finally, a big thank you to my husband Phill Turner and my family, for all their love and encouragement.

Make-up, Illustrations, and Words
Gary Cockerill
Make-up Assistants
Abbi Rose, Marijelle Moreno, Suzy Blackley, and Chloe Fennell
Clothes Stylist and Hair Design
Joey Bevan
Assistant Hair Stylist
Charlie Wilkinson
Photographer
Vikki Grant

Digital Operator
Karl Grant
Digital Retouching
James Bernasconi
Product Photographs
Tom Watson
Assistant to Gary Cockerill
Megan Flaherty
Portrait of Gary Cockerill (page 8 and endpapers)
Alan Strutt

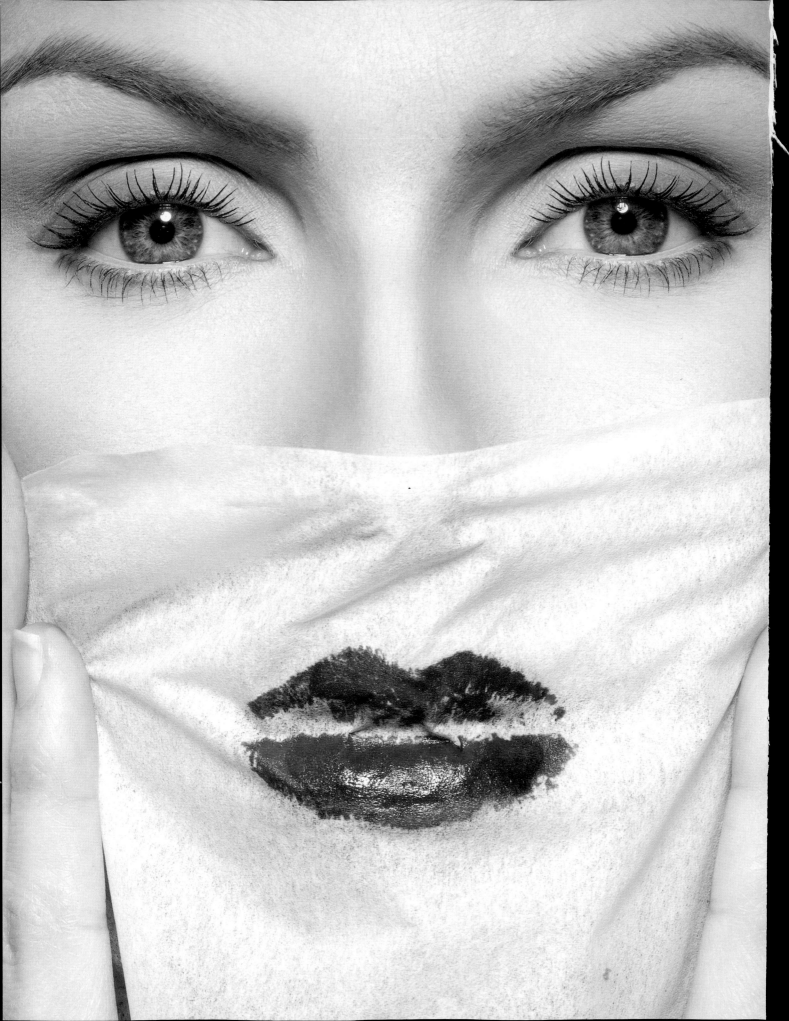

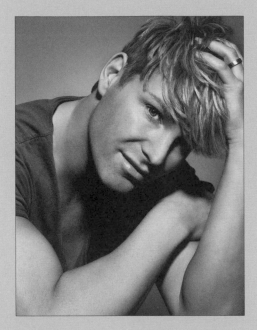

Gary Cockerill is one of the UK's most successful celebrity make-up artists with a repertoire of work spanning stage and screen, editorial, events, and advertising. Much sought after for his super-sexy, glamorous make-up style, Gary has an extensive client list that includes male and female stars of all ages—Kelly Brook, Martine McCutcheon, Jerry Hall, Eva Longoria, Honor Blackman, Isla Fisher, Katie Price, Rachel Hunter, Melanie Griffith, Rupert Everett, and David Beckham, to name a few. Gary's attention to detail and drive for perfection result in some of the most exquisite imagery. His philosophy—"external beauty promotes inner confidence"—means that he strives to make every client look and feel amazing.

He is a regular guest speaker and consultant for make-up brands on product development, and has had many roles as a brand ambassador. He is currently working on an exciting new color cosmetics collection for launch in 2016.

www.garycockerill.com